Subscribed to Thrive:
A Mental Health Resolve

By

Elijah Olla

ISBN:

978-1-965221-18-1 **(Paperback)**

978-1-965221-17-4 **(Hardback)**

Disclaimer

The unfolding tale of "DeCola" and the ensemble of characters within these pages spring from the realm of fiction, meticulously crafted to kindle awareness and dialogue around mental health. The narrative weaves through imaginary scenarios, not to mirror real-life individuals or particularized clinical practices but to illuminate the complexities of mental health and the criticality of crisis intervention.

The name "DeCola" is a fictional construct and does not represent or substitute for any real person or patient. This story, while having benefitted from the analytical touch of AI, is the brainchild of human creativity aimed at navigating the intricate subject of mental health. It doesn't claim to offer clinical solutions but seeks to foster a deeper understanding and appreciation for the integrated care mental wellness demands. The goal is to provide a conceptual understanding of certain aspects of mental health care as well as reflect the compelling need to consistently involve qualified and experienced professionals with proven minds at any stage of a mental health crisis. Suppose this tale succeeds in kindling a spark of awareness, encouraging one more individual to view mental health through a lens of empathy and understanding. In that case, the novel has fulfilled its purpose.

Dedication

Dedicated to all those who are concerned about mental health and are committed to making a difference.

I dedicate this book to my incredible editing team, AKDP. Your unwavering support, meticulous attention to detail, and dedication have made this journey possible. Thank you for bringing my vision to life.

About the Author

Driven by a profound passion for the holistic care of humanity, the author embraces the unique essence of each individual and the collective harmony of communities. His diverse academic journey includes Veterinary Science, Mental Health Science, Theology, Religious Studies, Computer Technology, Computer Networking and Computer Engineering, and Desktop Publishing. With over three and a half decades of dedicated experience across various sectors, he remains committed to advocating for peace and the betterment of mankind.

Contents

Introduction

DeCola's story is not just a tale; it is a deliberate walk through the murky waters of mental illness, where the specters of despair and isolation loom large. Yet, it is also a narrative brimming with the potential for breakthrough and transformation. DeCola, once trapped in the grips of mental turmoil, embarks on a quest not only for survival but for a profound sense of aliveness—a subscription to thrive in its most authentic essence.

In the heart of a world teeming with untold stories and silent struggles, "Subscribed to Thrive: A Mental Health Resolve" emerges as a vivid narrative tapestry, interwoven with the threads of resilience, hope, and the indomitable human spirit. At its core, this book is a testament to the journey of DeCola, a character whose life is a mirror to the complexities and tumultuous waves of mental health challenges.

This book is more than a collection of pages; it is a lighthouse for those navigating the shadowy paths of mental health difficulties. Identifying with DeCola, it is crafted to resonate with you and with anyone who finds themselves or their loved ones grappling with similar battles. Through De-Cola's eyes, we explore the intricate landscape of mental health, from its foundational significance in shaping our perceptions and experiences to the stealthy way it can unravel the fabric of our lives.

As DeCola delves deeper into understanding and confronting mental health conditions, a narrative unfolds that is rich in insights and revelations. These pages are imbued with the knowledge that mental health is not a destination but a journey—one that is punctuated with challenges yet abundant in opportunities for growth and renewal.

Imagine standing at the crossroads of humanity, where every path is intertwined with stories of struggle, self-pity, resilience, and the undying spirit of empathy. This book, a masterpiece of illustrated narratives, beckons you to step beyond the fences—whether you find yourself looking in from the outside of the walls of mental health crises or gazing out from within the confinements. It's a journey that transcends the boundaries of our individual experiences, inviting us to unite in our collective concern to ride on the storms of mental health.

Crafted with care and profound insight, the stories within these pages—brought to life through Elijah's variegated experience and the inspiring saga of DeCola—serve as a mirror reflecting the myriad facets of the human condition. This book is not merely a collection of experiences; it's a vibrant blend of life's highs and lows, its trials and triumphs, each panel and line infused with the essence of real-life encounters.

Woven into the fabric of this narrative is the symbolic story of DeCola, who traversed the rugged terrains of mental health challenges and emerged with stories of hope and triumph. These stories are not just anecdotes; they are altogether a beam of light that illuminates the shared path of human resilience, underscoring the universal truth that while each journey is unique, the pursuit of healing and wholeness is a collective human endeavor.

Empowerment is the cornerstone of "Subscribed to Live." DeCola's story is a clarion call to embrace self-care as well as support others in the struggle as an act of rebellion against the stigma and shadows that often shroud mental health. It champions the myriad of strategies available to fortify mental resilience, from the simplicity of daily routines that anchor us to the profound impact of lifestyle choices that nourish our minds and bodies. Moreover, it underscores the importance of seeking and embracing professional support as an integral component of a holistic approach to well-being.

For those who have ever felt the weight of the world's woes or the joy of a heart's uplift, this narrative is your clarion call. It's an invitation to explore the depths of empathy, to understand the intricacies of mental health not as a distant concept but as a reality that touches us all. Through Elijah's storytelling venture and healthcare experience spanning decades, interlaced with the concept of DeCola's mental adventure, this book emerges as a lighthouse of hope and understanding in a world often dimmed by ignorance and stigma.

"Subscribed to Thrive: A Mental Health Resolve" invites you to join DeCola to embark on a journey of self-discovery and transformation. It is an invitation to engage actively in the pursuit of well-being to embrace life with a renewed sense of purpose and joy. This book is not just a guide; it is a companion for those moments when the path seems uncertain and the journey daunting.

Why should you be compelled to read this book? Because within its pages lies the power to change perspectives, to break down the barriers that divide us, and to kindle a collective spirit of support and compassion. It's an exploration that promises not just to enlighten but to inspire action, to encourage conversations that bridge gaps, and to foster a community that stands united in the face of mental health challenges.

This book is your invitation to be part of something larger than yourself—a movement towards empathy, understanding, and public mutual support. Whether you're outside looking in or inside looking out, this narrative holds a place for you. It's a call to join hands, to share in the universal human experience, and to be part of the collective effort to illuminate the path towards mental wellness for all. Let this book be your gateway to a world where empathy reigns, where stories of courage and compassion light the way, and where every reader becomes a symbol of hope in the ongoing journey toward understanding and supporting mental health.

To you, like or unlike DeCola, to all who are mirrored or find a reflection of others they know in these pages, let this book be a guide toward a more informed, healthier, and happier existence. Embrace the journey, for in the very act of reading. You are taking the first step toward subscribing to a life where mental health is not just a resolve but a vibrant, lived reality. Welcome to "Subscribed to Thrive: A Mental Health Resolve."

The Quiet Before the Storm

In the gentle hum of everyday life, where dreams weave through the fabric of mundane routines, DeCola stood as an embodiment of silent resilience and unspoken aspirations. To the casual observer, DeCola was like any other, navigating the ebb and flow of daily existence with quiet determination. Mornings were greeted with the soft glow of dawn, the rhythmic pulse of the daily commute, and evenings wrapped in the comforting lull of familiar spaces. These were the threads that wove the tapestry of DeCola's youthful life, a life punctuated by occasional victories and fleeting joys that give color to daily ventures.

Yet, beneath the surface of this seemingly tranquil routine, subtle undercurrents whispered of a storm brewing in the depths. DeCola, with aspirations as vast as the night sky, harbored silent battles that went unnoticed in the hustle of life. Laughter came easy, and smiles were freely given, but in the quiet moments, when the world seemed to pause, a shadow lingered in DeCola's eyes—a reflection of the invisible weights carried within.

It started as a whisper, a faint murmur in the back of the mind, easily dismissed as the residue of a day too long or a night too short. The vibrant tapestry of dreams and aspirations seemed to dull ever so slightly as if a grey veil was gently being drawn across. The once invigorating routines began to feel like chains, binding DeCola to a cycle that seemed increasingly devoid of color.

Friends would ask, and DeCola would deflect, attributing the weary smile to the usual suspects—just a rough patch, a bad night's sleep, or the endless grind. "I'm just tired" became the refrain, a mask worn so often it almost felt true. After all, who wasn't tired in this whirlwind of existence? But this tiredness, this unrelenting fatigue, was a harbinger of the disruption to come, a subtle signal of the storm brewing beneath the calm facade.

In the quiet before the storm, life carried on, with DeCola at its helm, steering through the days with practiced ease. Yet, the undercurrents of strain grew stronger, the whispers louder, and the veil thicker. The world, once vibrant with the hues of dreams and the light of aspirations, now seemed to wane under the weight of an invisible force, setting the stage for a journey that would traverse the deepest valleys of the mind and soul.

Thus begins the tale of "Subscribed to Thrive: A Mental Health Resolve," a journey into the heart of darkness and back, guided by the light of resilience, hope, and an unwavering resolve to live. This is not just DeCola's story; it is a mirror reflecting the silent struggles many face, a motivation for those navigating the tumultuous seas of mental health, and a testament to the enduring strength of the human spirit.

Chapter 1: The Descent

Before the storm of mental adversity darkened his skies, DeCola was a symbol of youthfulness, fueled by an insatiable desire for achievement, his spirit adorned with the vibrant sails of hope and ambition. Within the boundless sea of life's opportunities, however, he found himself adrift, trapped by the invisible currents of societal norms and the daunting tides of personal goals. As the wheel of time turned, so did the fortunes in DeCola's voyage, with each successive wave bringing an onslaught of stressors that gradually began to wear down the pillars of his mental equilibrium.

The academic and professional arenas, once sources of exhilaration and purpose, transformed into a complex burden encompassing endless deadlines and demands, making each day a relentless battle against the surge of escalating stress. The sanctuary of the home, once a haven of tranquillity, was besieged by the unexpected storms of personal tragedy and the profound silence that ensued, leaving a void where once there was laughter and warmth. Financial burdens intricately entwined themselves into DeCola's daily concerns, their constricting embrace exacerbated by unforeseen expenses and the looming specter of financial instability.

Amidst these tumultuous waters, DeCola's once-luminous dreams began to dim, obscured by the gathering storm clouds of disenchantment and despair. The passionate quest for his dreams was supplanted by a grim struggle for mere survival, with each day becoming a monotonous echo of the one before, painting his world in increasingly desolate and restrictive hues.

During this chaos, the subtle murmurs of denial began to take root. DeCola, steadfast and unyielding, refused to acknowledge the encroaching shadows of mental exhaustion. Clinging to the belief that this was merely a transient rough patch, he rehearses this with determination, hoping to ward off the escalating unease. The concept of mental health struggles seemed alien, a plight reserved for others, not for DeCola, who was perceived as a bastion of strength by those around him.

Yet, this denial served as a double-edged sword. It propelled DeCola forward, albeit at a great cost. Isolation sneaked in secretly, rendering conversations superficial and social engagements increasingly scarce. His world contracted to the narrow confines of daily routines as the rich tapestry of his social life began to unravel at the edges.

The stigma associated with mental health, an invisible yet pervasive force in society, cast a long, chilling shadow over DeCola's psyche. Acknowledging his struggles felt tantamount to conceding defeat, exposing a vulnerability too profound to unveil in a society that often misinterprets mental health as a mere matter of determination rather than an essential aspect of overall well-being.

In this crucible of relentless stress, denial, and growing isolation, the cracks in DeCola's mental foundation deepened, setting the stage for a profound mental health crisis. It was a journey often undertaken in solitude, shrouded by the stigma that envelops mental health in obscurity, yet it also held the potential for enlightenment, recovery, and a rekindled determination to thrive.

In the core of DeCola's life, where the dawn's light casts a spectrum of hope across the sky and the night air carries whispers of dreams not yet realized, a silent narrative yearns for a voice. This is the tale of a youth, a bearer of tomorrow's promise, threading his path through the complex dance of maturation, cradled by the community's embrace.

For the families in DeCola's world, they stand as the bedrock of his voyage. Within the serenity of the home, members gathered around the dinner table and across the decorated scene of their backyards. They knit the initial strands of assurance and belonging into the essence of their young ones. Their affection serves as the directional support in navigating through tumults, and their belief in them acts as the lift beneath their wings.

The educational citadels within DeCola's realm, from schools to institutions, altogether emerge as a compass, steering the vessels of youthful intellects across the oceans of enlightenment and exploration. Within these halls, brimming with echoes of joy and the pursuit of knowledge, the youth are sculpted not solely in mind but in character as well. It is within these confines that seeds of understanding, innovation, and fortitude are sown, ensuring every young heart feels acknowledged, valued, and propelled.

To the dynamic entities and fervent collectives within DeCola, committed to the empowerment and evolution of the youth, their endeavors construct the framework upon which aspirations take shape. Through their initiatives and schemes, gateways to uncharted knowledge are unlocked, providing a spectrum of possibilities for the youth to sketch their destinies with bold hues of ambition and intent.

The fabric of DeCola's society, interwoven with myriad strands, is called upon to foster a culture of acceptance and backing. The triumphs of the youth to be exalted, their ventures supported, and a safety network of communal care established to embrace them in moments of stumble. It is within the symphony of collective action that DeCola's success finds its cadence.

And to the stewards of governance, the crafters of DeCola's structural edifice, their policies and foresight lay the foundation for the youth's expedition. Investments as the cornerstone of education, the refuge of mental health assistance, and the nurturing grounds of empowerment initiatives are imperative, nurturing an environment where every young spirit can bloom and blossom, unencumbered by the tangles of hardship.

Thus, DeCola's mental health journey illuminates the essence of warm collective support and communal dedication. Together, all represent the keepers of youth aspirations, the guides on their path, and the advocates of their achievements. For in their flourishing resides not only the future of DeCola but a legacy of hope and resilience that will resonate through generations.

Nonetheless, it is the inadequacies of DeCola's fortresses that nudge him towards the search for satisfaction. He eventually stumbled upon the deceptive allure of substance abuse. Its siren calls, promising a haven from his turmoil. The initial foray into this realm offered a semblance of relief, a temporary respite from his burdens, where the tumultuous seas of his inner turmoil calmed, and clarity seemed momentarily within reach and catastrophe looming.

However, what started as an occasional indulgence, seeking solace in the deceptive comfort of substances, quickly devolved into perilous wanderings, steering him ever closer to ruin. As substances assumed the roles of companions and navigators, DeCola's once-clear life map grew increasingly obscured. The attainable fulfillment he fervently chased was shrouded in a thick fog of dependency, each indulgence drawing the rope tighter around him, trapping him in a relentless cycle of consumption and craving, leaving his spirit weathered and withered by the repercussions.

In this pursuit of fleeting happiness, the impact on DeCola's mental health was both silent and profound. The very substances that promised a glimpse of serenity instead cast a gloom over his perception, eroding the bedrock of his mental health like relentless waves on a fragile shoreline. What began as an external quest for fulfillment devolved into an internal tempest, a mental health disaster threatening to engulf him.

In the shadowed realm of DeCola's mind, reality intertwines with the unseen variables. The seductive whispers of mental health voices craft a deceptive narrative, blending truth with illusion.

As DeCola navigated the turbulent waters of his mental health crisis, he reflected on a peculiar aspect of his experience: the distinct voices that seemed to communicate with him. These were not just any voices but ones that spoke in a manner deeply resonant with DeCola, utilizing the medium of poetry—a form of expression that had always captivated him. These ethereal voices, poetic in their cadence, offered him guidance, whispering directions and instructions that seemed to emerge from the fog of his mental turmoil. As he grappled with the complexities of his condition, these voices became a source of both intrigue and direction, weaving through his thoughts like threads of an unseen tapestry.

DeCola's connection to poetry, with its rich layers of meaning and emotion, made these auditory experiences particularly impactful. The voices, often clear and articulate, seemed to echo from the depths of his psyche, offering a form of communication that was both familiar and compelling. They spoke to him at moments of deep contemplation when the weight of his mental struggles pressed heavily upon his shoulders, providing a semblance of clarity amid the chaos.

However, as time passed and DeCola journeyed further into the labyrinth of his mental health crisis, he began to discern the true nature of these guiding whispers. He realized that not all the directives provided by these poetic voices were benevolent. Some, he discovered, were misleading, leading him down paths that only compounded his distress. Others were outright ruthless, suggesting actions and thoughts that were harmful to himself and potentially to others around him. This revelation was an unbearable contrast to the initial allure of the voices, unmasking a darker aspect of his mental struggle.

Despite recognizing the potentially deceptive and destructive nature of these instructions, DeCola found himself at times unable to resist their guidance. He acknowledged a profound vulnerability within himself, a susceptibility born from the depths of his suffering. This fragility made him more receptive to the voices, even when a part of him understood that their counsel was not to be trusted. The voices exploited this vulnerability, their poetic allure making it all the more difficult for him to dismiss them outright.

DeCola's introspection revealed a complex relationship with these auditory experiences. On one hand, they provided a form of companionship and guidance through the lonely and confusing landscape of his mental health crisis. On the other, they represented a dangerous element of his condition, capable of leading him astray with their seductive yet sometimes malevolent whispers.

This duality underscored the challenges DeCola faced as he sought to navigate his mental health crisis. The voices, with their poetic resonance, were a testament to the power of the mind to create experiences that are profoundly real and influential, for better or for worse. DeCola's struggle to discern and resist the more harmful aspects of these voices highlighted the importance of seeking and adhering to trusted forms of guidance and support as he worked to reclaim the narrative of his mental well-being.

DeCola remembered specific occasions as the nights steeped into tranquillity when a calm voice would recite poetry to him, an obscured companion under the cloak of darkness. Among these whispered verses was a promise below, a misleading camouflage of hope of a brighter life lying just beyond the horizon. This experience was DeCola's initial introduction to a world other than the one he was accustomed to. Yet, the introductory promise, veiled in poetic charm, unwittingly guided him further into the web of his mind, entangling him in layers of confusion, complicating his journey through the shadowed realms of mental strife:

"Beyond the earthly veil, your eyes could see through.

To silent whispers, your ears could be attuned.

Scents supernatural, your nose could perceive,

Besides your tongue, the taste could still be real.

By extraordinary touch, your flesh could align.

Beyond the visible, you could know, as you could be well known."

The poem spoke to DeCola in a language that transcended words, inviting him to explore realms beyond the physical, where senses are heightened and perceptions broadened. It offered a sense of connection to something greater, a reminder that there is more to existence than the material world can offer. In the depths of his struggle, this poem served as a reminder of the vastness of the human spirit and its ability to connect with the mysteries of the universe, providing a momentary escape from the confines of his mental turmoil.

This poetic encapsulation mirrors DeCola's journey into a world where the lines between reality and delusion blur, creating a narrative in which his perceptions are swayed by the internal dialogues shaped by his mental health struggles. These "seductive whispers" suggest the allure of these delusions, how they can seem convincingly real and preferable to the harsh realities of his condition. The "deceptive narrative" reflects the distorted reality in which DeCola lives, where everyday objects and interactions are imbued with meanings and threats that exist only in his mind.

The deceptive narrative spun by the "whispers of mental health voices" in DeCola's mind illustrates the profound challenge of discerning reality amidst the distortions of mental illness. This internal struggle not only exacerbates his disconnection from the external world but also impedes the path to recovery, creating a labyrinth of illusions that obscure the way forward.

His struggle with mental illness manifested in unusual behaviors, such as imposing irrational restrictions on his family, driven by delusions and hallucinations. These demands, ranging from prohibitions against certain colors to bizarre directives about clothing, highlight the depth of his detachment from reality. Such actions not only strained familial relationships but also alienated him further, creating a chasm that his loved ones struggled to bridge despite their devoted care and sacrifices.

The retreat of friends, once a constant presence in his life, underscores the impact of his deteriorating mental state on his social circle. His mistrust and misinterpretation of their intentions reveal a profound distortion in his perception of social interactions, pushing him into deeper isolation.

DeCola's neglect of personal hygiene and care is a stark indicator of the internal chaos wrought by his mental health crisis. The abandonment of routine self-care practices, such as bathing and maintaining his appearance, serves as a physical manifestation of his inner turmoil. His hair, once perhaps a point of pride, now remains unkempt, a tangled mass

– an evolved style that needs no special care, bereft of meticulous grooming habits, thus giving way to utter neglect, mirroring the disorder that dominates his psyche.

His vehement rejection of professional support and assistance, including matters of basic hygiene, signifies a fierce but faltering attempt to cling to independence. This resistance reflects a broader struggle against the vulnerability and perceived infantilization that comes with accepting help, highlighting the complex interplay of pride, fear, and despair in his battle with mental illness.

Even the outdoors, once a refuge and a source of joy through exercise, now feels fraught with danger. DeCola perceives threats in the glances and words of passersby, transforming what were once routine outings into gauntlets of perceived hostility.

DeCola's response to unfamiliar cars arriving near his home, particularly when they are positioned in such a way that they face his windows or door, is marked by a surge of impulsivity. This reaction is driven by a heightened sense of vulnerability and a perceived intrusion into his personal space. The sight of a vehicle oriented towards his living quarters triggers in him an urgent need to establish control over his immediate environment, compelling him to step out and confront the occupants.

These confrontations typically involve DeCola questioning the strangers with an intensity that belies the commonality of the situation—cars parked in public spaces within residential areas. He demands explanations for their presence, their intentions, and why they choose to position their vehicles in a manner that he finds provocative. To an outsider, these interactions seem unwarranted or excessive, given the benign nature of most such occurrences in public or semi-public spaces.

This pattern of behavior, however, escalates stress not only for DeCola but also for his family. Each impulsive reaction to perceived threats magnifies the atmosphere of tension within the household. His family caught between understanding DeCola's troubled state of mind and navigating the social ramifications of his public confrontations, finds themselves in a delicate balance. They must manage the immediate fallout of these incidents while also contending with the broader, more insidious impact of DeCola's actions on their collective mental well-being.

The underlying issue here extends beyond mere impulsive behavior; it is symptomatic of a deeper, unresolved anxiety that DeCola experiences concerning his safety and the sanctity of his home environment. This persistent state of hyper-vigilance not only exacerbates his stress levels but also casts a shadow of unease over his family, perpetuating a cycle of tension with apprehension that strains their resilience and coping mechanisms.

DeCola's isolation, compounded over a year, transformed him from a vibrant, friendly individual into a recluse lost in a "digital wilderness," detached from the tangible warmth of human connections. This digital realm, while vast and boundless, offered little solace or remedy to his growing sense of alienation. His once joyous demeanor, characterized by laughter and jokes, has been eclipsed by a profound withdrawal from the world around him.

Complicating his experience, DeCola frequently finds himself in the grip of intense fear, convinced that unseen adversaries are infiltrating his digital life. His paranoia extends even to mundane activities such as answering phone calls, fearing that these too might be conduits for those he believes seek to harm him.

Television, once a source of entertainment and relaxation, has become another arena for his torment as DeCola became convinced that personal messages and calls are being directed at him through the screen, further feeding his sense of persecution. The concern which often made him anxious and restless. During a solitary evening dedicated to the enjoyment of a football match, a seemingly mundane activity took an unexpected turn. Seated before his television, he was engrossed in the game when a moment of perplexing audio intrusion shattered the normalcy. The commentator, amid the usual play-by-play, appeared to veer off script, articulating his name with unsettling clarity and coupling it with a direct threat of harm. This bizarre and alarming incident prompted him to rush out of the room, a blend of confusion and fear propelling his steps as he sought his father to relay what had transpired.

To an outsider, the claim might have bordered on the incredulous, easily dismissed as a figment of an overactive imagination or misinterpretation. However, within the confines of his family, this incident was not hastily brushed aside. They were intimately acquainted with the silent battles he had been waging, the mental health challenges that cast long shadows over his everyday experiences. This familiarity with his struggles lent a different hue to the episode, infusing it with a gravity that might have otherwise been absent.

The family, well aware of the deceptive manifestations of psychological distress, understood that what might seem fantastical or improbable to others could very well be a vivid reality to him. The incident sparked concerns, raising questions about the nature of his experiences and the possible worsening of his mental health condition. It underscored the pressing need for attentive care and the exploration of therapeutic interventions, aiming to navigate the complex labyrinth of his mental well-being and ensure his safety against the backdrop of his unique perceptual experiences.

His solution, to retreat further into his world with the aid of headphones, listening only to familiar music, serves as a barrier to keep the imagined aggressors at bay.

In moments of acute distress, he reaches out to the authorities, his voice trembling as he reports what he perceives as malicious intrusions into his devices. He articulates a narrative of being pursued, a tale where shadowy figures lurk behind screens, orchestrating a campaign of intimidation that leaves him feeling profoundly vulnerable.

To DeCola, these episodes are not mere figments of imagination but palpable threats that disrupt his peace and perpetuate a state of constant vigilance. The digital realm, a space that should offer connection and information, morphs into a battlefield in his mind, where every ping, every unsolicited notification, is interpreted as a harbinger of a more sinister plot against him.

However, to those who share his life and home, this pattern of behavior is a manifestation of unwarranted paranoia.

Socially, DeCola has summarily receded into a shell of suspicion and withdrawal. The vibrant connections he once maintained with family and friends, the very relationships that once enriched his life, have now faded into the background.

They observe these recurrent episodes with a mix of concern and helplessness, recognizing a stark discrepancy between DeCola's perceived dangers and the reality of their secure, mundane digital interactions. To them, the absence of tangible evidence points not to a well-concealed conspiracy but to the troubling specter of DeCola's mental health struggles casting long shadows over his perception of reality.

The connection of DeCola's palpable dread against the backdrop of his loved ones' understanding of his arbitrary paranoia paints a complex picture. It highlights the isolating nature of mental health challenges, where the afflicted individual's experiences, so vivid and distressing, often remain invisible or incomprehensible to those around them. This divergence in perceptions not only underscores the subjective nature of fear and safety but also the critical need for empathy, support, and professional intervention in navigating the labyrinth of mental health.

DeCola later attributed his psychological challenges to the profound impact of internalizing a compelling poetic message he had previously encountered, which had significantly disrupted his cognitive processes. He realized that the remnants of this poetic message were persistently echoing within his mind, compelling him to reflect on them involuntarily. This constant rumination meant that he was subconsciously governed by the enigmatic words that had been permanently etched into his consciousness. As someone naturally inclined towards the allure of rhythm and rhyme, DeCola perceived the influence of an invisible force that seemed to amplify the message's impact, intricately interlacing its core meaning more deeply within his thought patterns.

This insidious process not only intensified the message's resonance but also subtly manipulated his mental landscape, further embedding its essence into his psyche.

The rhythmic haunting beauty becomes vessels for these deceits, weaving a chronicle that transcends the mundane to touch upon the divine yet masks the treacherous undercurrents beneath:

"Beyond the earthly veil, your eyes could see through" speaks to the allure of hidden truths, promising insight beyond the reach of ordinary perception. Yet, this vision, granted by the unseen stimulus, is a double-edged sword, offering enlightenment at the cost of disconnection from the tangible world.

"To silent whispers, your ears could be attuned" hints at the seduction of secret knowledge, the enticing call of voices that offer an escape from solitude. These whispers, however, carry a weight, binding the listener to a chorus of confusion and doubt.

"Scents supernatural, your nose could perceive," suggests an elevation above the earthly, a promise of purity untainted by the earthly. But this sanctity is a mirage, leading one away from the grounding scents of life's reality.

"Besides your tongue, the taste could still be real" implies a mysterious taste beyond the capabilities of the physical taste buds, suggesting an otherworldly experience luring one away from the visible world.

"By extraordinary touch, your flesh could align" implies a transformation, a redefinition of self through an invisible caress. Yet, this alignment strays from the essence of human experience, distancing one from the warmth of human touch.

"Beyond the visible, you could know, as you could be well known," which seemingly beckons DeCola to become a celebrity, is a clear illusion of his mental faculties.

The poem apparently captures the intoxicating blend of the senses heightened beyond normalcy. But in this extraordinary entanglement, the lines between the real and the imagined blur, leading to disorienting spirals.

The overall message of the poems delves deeper into the deception, challenging the very foundations of perception. It speaks of a heightened awareness that transcends the physical, suggesting an elevated existence. Yet, beneath the facade of such a transcendence lies the stark reality of isolation, a detachment from the communal fabric of life.

The perceived poetic verses, with their lyrical allure, mirror the deceptive nature of the voices that haunt DeCola's mind. They promise a realm of feeling "high", of senses attuned to the whispers of a world beyond. But this promise is a figment, a beautifully woven illusion that ensnares the mind, leading one away from the anchor of reality into the depths of a solitary struggle.

As DeCola relentlessly pondered upon the musical game of words, the stark contrast between the promised elevation and the underlying deception becomes clear. The verses, while enchanting, serve as a reminder of the treacherous path that mental health voices can lead one down—a path where the extraordinary becomes a veil, obscuring the essential truths of human connection, blurring the inherent value of navigating the world through senses anchored in reality.

As time passed, the allure of that initial high became a distant memory, an elusive feeling that DeCola chased with increasing desperation. The more he indulged in enhancing substances, the more desensitized he became to the effects of the weed, leading him down a dangerous path in search of something stronger, something that could reignite the extinguished flames of the earliest experience.

This quest for a greater high led DeCola to darker corners, where more potent drugs promised the intensity of sensation he so craved. Each step further into the abysmal world was a step away from the person he once was as the drugs began to weave their destructive web through the very fabric of his being.

Unrecognized by DeCola, each stimulating substance he experimented with makes the toll upon his mind and body grow heavier. The drugs, once a source of solace, became architects of ruin, slowly eroding his mental clarity and physical health. The intelligent and vibrant young man, who once faced the world with bright eyes and boundless potential, was gradually overshadowed by the specter of addiction.

The realization of his predicament was becoming too late, as DeCola found himself trapped in a cycle of dependency that was as relentless as it was unforgiving. The once occasional escape transformed into a dire necessity, a master to which DeCola was a slave. The dreams he harbored, the aspirations that once fueled his spirit, were now casualties of a war he waged within himself, a war where every battle left him weaker and fractured than before.

DeCola's story serves as a poignant reminder of the insidious nature of drug addiction, the major cause of pain and loss it inflicts not just on the individual but on the interrelationship with theirs.

Incredibly, DeCola became emotionally estranged from his family as he did not see anything wrong with him. Rather, he is convinced that the world, including his family, is entangled in a web of envy and competition, fueling his being misunderstood, accounting for continued confrontation, warranting an endless cycle of discord, disputes, conflict and hatred, the universal warfare that plagues humanity. He is baffled and disheartened by the world's inability to see that visionary minds like his own are the key to halting the rapid decline and impending self-annihilation of civilization. This, of course, is the overwhelming effects of the self-prescribed potent drugs upon his heavy-laden mind.

Repeated forgetfulness - the tendency to lose track of usual routines, including burning his self-cooked food aside from misplacing his keys on a regular basis represents another dimension of his frustration. The apprehensive fear of being assisted, considering the perceived threats of family members, has a ripple effect on DeCola's interactions. The aggression he feels from the world around him is, at times,

redirected towards those who mean no harm, casting inno-
cent individuals as worthy recipients of his bottled-up frustration and anger.

In the stillness that envelops DeCola's home, an extraordinary scene unfolds with a frequency that both bewilders
and captivates his family. From the vantage point of his window, one that frames the green expanse of the garden in a
picturesque embrace, DeCola engages in an activity that
transcends the boundaries of the ordinary. It is here, amid the
rustle of leaves and the gentle sway of branches, that he
claims to converse with the avian inhabitants that frequent
this natural haven. His family, often silent witnesses to these
interactions, watch with a blend of astonishment and intrigue
as he articulates what he perceives to be the nuanced dialects
of bird language.

This communion with the feathered creatures is not
merely an exchange of pleasantries or the sharing of the garden's tranquillity. DeCola assigns a more profound, albeit
mystifying, significance to these encounters. He believes
that among the myriad of birds that perch and flutter before
him, certain ones bear the heavy mantle of being emissaries
dispatched by unseen adversaries. These birds, distinguished

33

by signs perceptible only to DeCola, are labeled as the avian vanguards of evil forces.

When such a bird lands within his domain, the serene scene is abruptly disrupted. DeCola, convinced of the bird's sinister purpose, responds with an intensity that starkly contrasts the usual peace of the garden. He employs loud, forceful vocalizations, a cacophony of human sound aimed at repelling these feathered harbingers of ill-intent. This ritual of expulsion, witnessed by his family, adds layers of complexity to their understanding of DeCola's world—a world where the lines between the seen and unseen, the known and the mysterious, blur intriguingly.

For his family, these episodes are more than mere quirks of behavior. They are windows into the depths of DeCola's psyche, hinting at a rich inner life teeming with narratives and beliefs that defy conventional understanding. Each incident of communication or confrontation with the birds weaves into the larger tapestry of DeCola's existence, challenging those around him to expand the boundaries of their empathy and comprehension.

The landscape of DeCola's life, viewed through the lens of his troubled mind, paints a deeply distressing picture. The convergence of neglected self-care eroded social bonds, pervasive suspicion, and an environment perceived as overtly hostile encapsulates a profound struggle, one that envelops DeCola in a ceaseless cycle of despair and aggression, leaving him entangled in a reality where solace and safety feel perpetually out of reach.

The disappointment and emotional turmoil experienced by DeCola's parents was profound and heart-wrenching. Imagine the immense sorrow that enveloped them as their son, plagued by the cruel distortions of mental illness, denied their very essence as his parents. Their once cherished memories, the bonds forged from his first breath, his first steps, and his words, were all suddenly invalidated by his delusional conviction of belonging to an entirely different family.

The shock of this denial sent waves of disbelief through their hearts, a piercing pain that perhaps felt akin to mourning the loss of a child still alive yet unreachable. Each denial from DeCola was like a blow to the very foundation of their family, crumbling the hopes and dreams they had nurtured for their son. The confusion and helplessness likely consumed their every thought as they grappled with the reality that the child they raised and loved with every fiber of their being could no longer see them as his pillars of support and love.

His parents' expressions, a harrowing blend of sorrow and disbelief, seemed to evaporate into the void of DeCola's unwavering delusion. The tears that welled in his mother's eyes, each a silent testament to years of love and sacrifice, went unnoticed by him. His father's enduring composure, crumbling under the weight of his son's denial, was met with nothing but indifference.

DeCola stood before them, enveloped in an aura of misguided certainty, impervious to the emotional turmoil that his prevailing world conjured. It was as if the very fabric of their familial bond, once strong and nurturing, had been shredded in DeCola's distorted reality. The poignant scene, ripe with the rawness of unreciprocated anguish, painted a stark picture of a son lost to his mind, leaving his parents to grapple with the shadow of the child they once knew.

In his parents' hearts, a relentless storm of grief and loss raged, tempered only by flickers of hope that someday, their son might find his way back to them, back to the truth of his origins and the unwavering love of his true family.

Amidst this emotional turbulence, their reactions were a complex intermingling of despair, anger, and an unyielding desire to reclaim their son from the clutches of his mental torment. The constant battle between wanting to confront his delusions head-on and the fear of further alienating him likely waged a silent war within them. The longing to see a glimmer of recognition in his eyes, to hear him utter "mom" or "dad" with the warmth and affection of yesteryears, became a distant yearning overshadowed by the stark reality of his illness.

Amid the profound heartache that often fills the room, DeCola remained detached, his conviction unshaken by the visible despair etched on his parents' faces. His words usually slice through the heavy domestic silence with a cold precision in outright denial of his legitimate family: "I know you are upset because the truth about the identity of my real parents, which you have hidden from me since childhood, is no longer shrouded in secrecy." To DeCola, his actual parents are mere impostors, which is the baseline.

His vigilance was constant, a strained string never allowed to slacken, for fear that even the most benign offerings of food and drink were laced with venom by those he could no longer trust. The very family that yearned to envelop him in their care was seen through his distorted gaze as nothing more than double-faced actors, their genuine concern masked by the roles of covert adversaries. This harrowing dance of doubt led him to scrutinize every morsel, every sip, for signs of betrayal, an exhausting ritual that only deepened his isolation.

Unable to fathom the cruel irony of being besieged by those he believed should be his sanctuary, DeCola found himself entangled in an enigmatic world, a labyrinth with no discernible exit. His perceived impotence against these formidable, shadowy forces that seemed to manipulate his reality from just beyond reach left him perpetually on edge. This ever-present tension manifested in bouts of irritability and aggression, a defensive armor against an onslaught of deceptive foes, leaving those around him bewildered and hurt by the unprovoked outbursts.

In this tragic narrative, DeCola's struggle was not just with the phantoms of his mind but with the heart-wrenching disconnect from the very essence of human connection— trust and the warmth of familial love, now alien concepts that he could neither grasp nor return.

In the tangle of DeCola's mind, hallucinations warp the fabric of his reality, creating a multisensory ordeal that is as convincing as it is isolating. He sees apparitions that flicker at the edges of his vision, shadowy figures that appear with startling clarity one moment and vanish the next, leaving him in a constant state of vigilance. These spectral entities, with their menacing whispers, the silence with ominous threats and commands, their voices are as real to him as those of flesh and blood.

The air around DeCola is often tainted with inexplicable odors that assault his senses – the metallic tang of blood that seems to hang thickly in the air or the acrid scent of burning those hints at unseen destruction. These smells envelop him, an invisible yet overpowering cloak of dread that no one else seems to notice or acknowledge.

Touch, too, becomes a traitor as phantom sensations grip him; the brush of an unseen hand or the push of an invisible force that nudges him towards actions he resists with all his might. The tactile experiences, devoid of any visible source, are as bewildering as they are frightening, complicating his disrupted senses.

Apparently, the most profound aspect of DeCola's trials is the stark disconnect between his vivid experiences and the dismissal by those around him. His earnest attempts to share his reality, to seek validation or understanding, are met with skepticism or outright denial. The people he once trusted, whose perceptions of the world he had shared, now refute the very essence of his experiences. This dismissal, this refusal to acknowledge the intensity and authenticity of what he sees, hears, smells, and feels, deepens his sense of alienation.

DeCola's disappointment was intense, a heavy cloak of disillusionment that weighed on him. The chasm between his reality and that of others seems impossible, rendering him a stranger in a world that refuses to see through his eyes. The loneliness of this existence, where every sense betrays the validity of his experiences, is constantly challenged, is a silent battle he wages, longing for understanding in a world that seems content to dismiss the profound depth of his turmoil.

The physical toll of his predicament is starkly evident. DeCola's once healthy physique has withered away, the result of significant weight loss and a stark neglect of personal hygiene.

In the middle of his mental health crisis, DeCola's room stood as a silent witness to the tumult raging within him. Once a refuge of comfort and personal expression, it had transformed into a stark emblem of his inner turmoil.

The walls, previously adorned with vibrant posters and artwork that spoke of DeCola's passions and dreams, were now bare, their emptiness mirroring the void he felt inside. Dust gathered on surfaces that once gleamed, a physical manifestation of the neglect that had seeped into every aspect of his life. The air hung heavy, stagnant with the weight of unspoken sorrows and the echoes of solitary days and nights.

In one corner lay a pile of unwashed clothes, a chaotic jumble of fabrics that seemed to mirror the disorder in De-Cola's mind. Each garment, once chosen with care to express his unique style, now lay forgotten, a testament to how the vibrancy of his spirit had been dimmed.

The bed, unmade and shrouded in crumpled sheets, bore the imprint of countless hours spent in restless contemplation or escape into fitful sleep. It had become less a place of rest and more a raft adrift on the stormy seas of DeCola's thoughts, a refuge from the relentless surge of anxiety and despair.

Scattered across the floor were notebooks and pens, remnants of DeCola's once fervent creativity. Pages filled with half-formed thoughts and sketches lay abandoned, symbols of projects and dreams halted mid-flight by the paralyzing grip of his mental anguish.

A thin layer of dust coated the once-lively bookshelf, each book a reminder of DeCola's love for learning, poems, and exploration, now untouched, their stories and knowledge locked away just like the parts of DeCola that he could no longer reach.

In this room, the very air seemed to whisper of loss and longing, each object a relic of life paused, each silence a cry for understanding and relief. It was within these walls that DeCola's struggle reached its crescendo, a poignant chapter in the biography of a young man fighting to find his way back to himself amidst the shadows of a mental health crisis.

In the intricate tapestry of DeCola's mental health journey, moments of unfounded laughter and sudden, unprovoked anger stood out like erratic stitches, drawing attention to the complexity of his internal struggle. These spontaneous bursts of emotion, disconnected from the immediate reality around him, were poignant indicators of the turmoil churning beneath the surface.

DeCola's laughter, often erupting in the absence of humor, was a curious spectacle. It was laughter without warmth, a mechanical mimicry of joy that never quite reached his eyes. This inexplicable giggling or smiling would emerge at the most inappropriate moments, leaving those around him perplexed. To an observer, it might have seemed as if DeCola was privy to some private joke, an unseen source of amusement. However, this laughter was not a reflection of joy but rather an involuntary response, a surface ripple over deeper, unseen currents of distress. It was as if his mind, tangled in the web of his crisis, occasionally fired misdirected signals, manifesting in these ungrounded expressions of hilarity.

Simultaneously, DeCola's demeanor could shift dramatically, his face clouding over with sudden anger, as swift and inexplicable as a storm appearing on a clear day. This anger was not directed at anyone or sparked by any discernible provocation. Instead, it seemed to well up from a reservoir of frustration and confusion that DeCola himself could not fully comprehend or articulate. The absence of a visible trigger only added to the enigma, painting a vivid picture of the internal chaos that DeCola grappled with.

These contrasting emotional outbursts were emblematic of the dissonance within DeCola's psyche, a stark reminder of the invisible battle he waged daily. The laughter and anger, seemingly without cause, were manifestations of the deeper disarray, the silent scream of a mind in turmoil. They underscored the unpredictable nature of mental health struggles, where the external signs often belie the complexity of the internal experience.

For DeCola, these unbidden expressions of emotion were both confusing and isolating, adding layers of complexity to his interactions and his self-perception. They served as constant, jarring reminders of the distance between his internal experience and the world around him, highlighting the profound challenge of navigating a path to recovery amidst the shifting sands of his mental state.

It is a cautionary tale that echoes the silent scream of dreams deferred and potentially destroyed, a stark warning to those who stand at the crossroads where unbridled curiosity meets inevitable consequences.

Chapter 2: The Struggle Within

Following his mental breakdown, DeCola's journey was essentially transformed into a complex quest for something elusive, namely, trust. The vibrant tapestry of his youth, once rich with the colors of confidence and ambition, had vanished as a mirage, shadowed by the specters of doubt and betrayal that often accompany mental health struggles.

In the aftermath of his breakdown, trust for DeCola became akin to a mythical treasure hidden within a labyrinth, guarded by the many-headed hydra of his fears and insecurities. Each head represented a different challenge: the fear of vulnerability, the sting of past disappointments, the echo of his inner critic—all intertwining, making the path to trust a daunting one.

DeCola found himself in a world where every interaction was a potential battleground, every extended hand possibly another mirage in the desert of his isolation. The ease with which he once navigated social waters had vanished, replaced by a cautious dance, a perpetual assessment of risks versus rewards. The instinctual human craving for connection was now tempered by a learned hesitance, a protective shield forged in the fires of his past experiences.

His attempts to reach out, to forge bonds anew, were often marred by the specter of his breakdown, a silent guard that cast long shadows over potential connections. Conversations became minefields, where words had to be weighed and measured lest they reveal too much, or worse, not enough. The fear of being misunderstood, of having his experiences trivialized or dismissed, loomed large, turning trust into a distant star, visible yet seemingly out of reach.

Yet, within this struggle, DeCola's resilience began to shimmer through the cracks. Each small victory, every moment of genuine understanding shared with another, became a beacon, guiding him through the fog. The quest for trust, though fraught with challenges, also became a journey of self-discovery, a slow reclamation of the parts of himself lost in the storm of his mental health crisis.

In this new chapter of his life, DeCola's struggle for trust became not just about finding others to believe in but about rediscovering faith in himself. It was about learning to trust his voice again, to acknowledge his worth and to embrace the vulnerability that comes with genuine connections. This quest, marked by both setbacks and small triumphs, unfolded as a testament to the enduring human spirit's capacity for healing, growth, and the eventual rekindling of trust in a world that once seemed devoid of it.

DeCola's Quest for Trust

For DeCola, trust within his family became as elusive as a mirage in a desert, a desired oasis that seemed to recede with every step he took toward it. The root of this growing chasm lay in a tapestry of misunderstandings and unspoken grievances that had woven itself over time. Conversations that should have been bridged became walls, with every missed opportunity for open dialogue adding another brick.

In the rare moments when DeCola attempted to share the whirlwind of his thoughts and feelings, his words often fell on ears that, though well-meaning, were tuned to a different frequency. His attempts at vulnerability were met with responses that, although intended to comfort, felt dismissive of the depth of his turmoil. Phrases like "Just cheer up" or "It's all in your head" became common refrains, inadvertently minimizing his struggle and widening the gap of misunderstanding.

Family gatherings, once a source of warmth and laughter, turned into minefields for DeCola. The light-hearted banter that danced around the room seemed to skirt the edges of his inner chaos, never quite touching the core of his experience. His smiles became masks, and his laughter, a well-rehearsed script to play the part expected of him, left him feeling more isolated in their midst.

The cumulative effect of these dynamics was a fortress around DeCola's heart, with anxiety, the drawbridge that he found increasingly difficult to lower. The fear of being misunderstood or, worse, dismissed became a guard at the gates, challenging the intentions of those who sought to enter.

In this landscape where trust seemed an unattainable dream, DeCola found himself adrift, longing for a haven where his voice could be heard, his feelings validated, and his experiences acknowledged. The journey to rebuild that trust within his family promised to be a challenging one, requiring not just the mending of bridges but the construction of new ones, built on the pillars of empathy, patience, and genuine understanding.

He then began to perceive an insensitivity and lack of understanding in everyone around him, feeling besieged by what he believes to be deceitful malevolent figures akin to invaders from another realm. In his eyes, there's no flaw within him; rather, he's convinced of a sudden, unprovoked betrayal by even his closest kin, attributing their distance not to any fault of his own but to jealousy of his remarkable intellect. DeCola begins to see himself as a rightful leader, perhaps a president or prime minister of a utopian nation, baffled and hurt by the skepticism and wary glances that meet his bold affirmations. To him, his potential is undeniable, yet he stands alone, misunderstood in his solitary conviction.

DeCola's journey through the fog of his mental turmoil was heartbreakingly lonely. Each gesture of support from his loved ones twisted into menacing threats by the specters of his mind. Every outstretched hand, every comforting word was perceived as a sinister ploy, a cunning trap laid with the intent to harm him for reasons unfathomable to his tormented psyche. He viewed the world through a lens darkened by despair, its every corner shadowed by malevolence, pushing him to the brink of contemplating the abyss of forgetfulness where no one could reach him, haunted by the belief that there was no action potent enough to deflect the barrage of undeserved hate.

DeCola's story is a nuanced exploration of the complexities that often intertwine within the fabric of mental health, trust, and familial relationships. As a young man, he found himself trapped in the throes of a mental health crisis, a journey that is deeply personal and fraught with challenges. His struggle with trust, particularly in the context of his family, is symbolic of the broader challenges he faced when navigating mental health issues within the dynamics of close relationships. At the core of DeCola's struggle was the dichotomy between the innate human need for connection and the fear of vulnerability that accompanies the admission of not being okay. Mental health crises can often feel isolating, creating a chasm between the individual and the outside world. For DeCola, this chasm was widened by a fear of judgment, misunderstanding, or the potential for his struggles to be minimized. This fear was not unfounded; societal stigmas surrounding mental health can infiltrate even the most loving of families, creating an environment where individuals may feel hesitant to share their true feelings. Trust, a fundamental element of any relationship, becomes particularly pivotal during a mental health crisis. For DeCola, his reluctance to trust his family with the depths of his struggles was twofold. Firstly, there was the concern of adding emotional burdens to his loved ones, a common fear among those suffering. Many individuals amid a mental health crisis worry about the impact their struggles might have on their loved ones, preferring to bear the weight alone rather than distribute it amongst those they care about. Secondly, there was the fear of not being truly heard or understood.

Misunderstandings about mental health, even among well-meaning family members, can lead to responses that, while intended to be supportive, may feel dismissive or inadequate to the individual in crisis. Phrases like "your brain is playing up" can deepen the sense of isolation and misunderstanding, making the prospect of opening even more daunting. The dynamics of familial relationships also play a significant role in this struggle. Each family has its unique communication patterns, history, and way of dealing with challenges. For DeCola, the existing dynamics within his family might have made it more challenging to explore sensitive topics or to feel confident that his experiences would be met with empathy and understanding rather than judgment or denial. In navigating his mental health crisis, DeCola's journey was not just about seeking help but also about bridging the gap of understanding within his family. It involved a delicate balance of self-advocacy and vulnerability, educating his loved ones about his experiences while also learning to trust in their capacity to support him. This process is rarely linear and is often marked by setbacks and breakthroughs alike. Ultimately, DeCola's story sheds light on the broader conversation about mental health, trust, and family dynamics. It underscores the importance of open communication, education, and empathy in navigating these complex waters. For families and individuals alike, understanding and addressing mental health challenges requires patience, compassion, and an ongoing commitment to learning and growth.

In a moment that left DeCola's real parents utterly speechless, he starts to confront his parents with a chilling accusation borne from his delusions. He questioned their identity with a haunting intensity, dismissing his mother's heartfelt affirmation of him as her beloved son as a mere facade. With a glare laden with scorn, DeCola unleashed a torrent of disbelief, declaring them mere impostors, stand-ins, paid off by his "true" father, who he claimed was a former President of the United States, embroiled in political turmoil. He spun a tale of tragic loss and high-stakes conspiracy, painting his actual parents as mere guardians appointed after his "purported" mother's dramatic assassination by the political rivals of his "acclaimed" father. DeCola wove a narrative of secret millions paid out for his care by his "asserted" protective father, to safeguard him, the sum of which was mismanaged by his parents he branded impostors. As the sole heir to his "millionaire father", he was supposed to be a young millionaire were it not for the wasteful impostors'. As this bewildering assertion hung in the air, his father was struck with astonishment while his mother, overwhelmed by the depth of his delusion, wept uncontrollably, her tears a silent testament to the profound heartache of watching her son drift further into his own fabricated reality.

In the haunting melody that DeCola weaved, his voice trembled with the weight of unseen chains, his words painting the stark landscape of his troubled mind. The song, a poignant confession of his distorted reality, echoed with the sorrow of misplaced belonging.

"Hired mummy cool, borrowed daddy cool," he sang, his voice a blend of defiance and despair as if each word was a step further away from the arms that once cradled him. "Don't you cry? Your pampered son will soon go home," the melody dipped, a tender plea wrapped in the confusion of his delusions, hinting at the love he once knew but could no longer grasp.

DeCola's struggle with trusting his friends during his mental health crisis is a profound aspect of his journey, highlighting the intricate interplay between personal vulnerability, societal perceptions of mental health, and the dynamics of friendship. His challenges in this area were multi-faceted, rooted in both internal and external factors that influenced his ability to confide in and rely on his friends. One of the primary barriers DeCola faced was the fear of being misconstrued. Mental health issues can be deeply personal and complex, and there's often a worry that others won't fully grasp the depth or nature of one's experience. DeCola was concerned that his friends, despite their best intentions, might not understand the intricacies of his struggles or the severity of his feelings. This fear was compounded by the common societal misconceptions about mental health, where emotional or psychological challenges are often oversimplified or stigmatized. DeCola also worried about how his revelations might alter the dynamics of his friendships. There's often a fear that once you expose your vulnerabilities, friends might treat you differently—either by walking on eggshells around you, changing the nature of your interactions, or, in the worst-case scenario, withdrawing their friendship altogether.

For DeCola, the value he placed on these relationships made the risk of potential change daunting. Integral to DeCola's reluctance to open up was the anxiety about burdening his friends with his troubles. He was acutely aware of the challenges and stresses his friends faced in their own lives and was hesitant to add to their load. This is a common concern among those experiencing mental health issues, where the individual's empathy for others paradoxically becomes a barrier to seeking support. DeCola's hesitance may have also been influenced by past experiences where his openness about personal struggles was met with rejection, dismissal, mischievous gossip, or inadequate responses. Such experiences can leave lasting impressions, making it difficult to approach others for fear of repeated hurt or disappointment. DeCola's struggle was further complicated by prevailing social norms and expectations around masculinity and emotional expression.

Societal pressures often dictate a certain level of composure, particularly among men, discouraging the expression of vulnerability or emotional distress. For DeCola, these cultural expectations might have served as an additional barrier to seeking support, fueling concerns about how his honesty might be perceived or judged by his peer group. In facing these challenges, DeCola's journey encapsulates the delicate balance between the human need for connection and the fears that can inhibit it.

Trust, especially in the context of mental health, involves more than just the act of sharing—it's about believing in the capacity of others to respond with empathy, under-standing, and support. For DeCola, overcoming these hur-dles with his friends required not only courage and vulnera-bility on his part but also a conducive environment where such openness is met with kindness and acceptance.

In the realm of DeCola's relationships, hope flickered like a candle in the wind. Trust, once freely given, now re-quired an effort to entrust himself unto others. Each attempt to connect was shadowed by the fear of misunderstanding, of not being seen or heard in the true depth of his struggle. The simple act of reaching out became fraught with the pos-sibility of rejection, turning each social interaction into a high-stakes gamble with his vulnerable heart on the line.

In the midst of his mental health crisis, DeCola encoun-tered profound difficulties in placing his trust within his community, a reflection of the broader challenges many face in reconciling mental health complexities with community life. This struggle was deeply rooted in a mix of societal prej-udices, the nature of communal support mechanisms, and DeCola's battle with vulnerability and the stigma surround-ing mental health. For DeCola, falling into depression more often is attributable to his overwhelming isolation.

Thus, DeCola grappled with the widespread stigma attached to mental health issues, a stigma that permeated his community and society at large. The cloud of misunderstanding and prejudice that often hangs over mental health led to a real fear for DeCola — a fear of being labeled, judged, or even ostracized by those around him. These concerns weren't unfounded; they stemmed from the harsh realities of how mental health is frequently misunderstood and stigmatized in various social circles.

DeCola's apprehension went beyond just the stigma; he was acutely aware of how quickly personal matters could become the subject of public discourse within close-knit communities. The prospect of his mental health struggles becoming fodder for gossip or speculative conversations was a significant barrier to seeking support locally. This fear of public exposure, of his deepest vulnerabilities being laid bare for communal scrutiny, compounded the challenges DeCola faced in his journey toward healing, adding a complex layer to his reluctance to engage with community-based support systems.

DeCola stands amidst the community he believes has forsaken its duty, a society that, in his eyes, should have been a stronghold of protection, especially for the vulnerable youth. He is bewildered and deeply disheartened by the collective dismissal of the sinister undercurrents he perceives— the evil forces at play, leaving behind a trail of chaos and the disgusting odor of bloodshed that only he seems to experience.

His frustration boils over as he confronts the stark reality of his isolation; he alone bears the burden of vigilance against these hidden threats. The community's dismissal of his warnings, the branding of his acute awareness as a mere oddity, cuts deep. DeCola feels stigmatized and ostracized for his heightened perception of his unique insight into the dangers that lurk within their midst. This betrayal, this failure of collective empathy and understanding, renders the community untrustworthy in his eyes.

"Why is my voice the only one raised in alarm?" He questions, his despair tinged with doubt. "How can they not see? Are they deliberately ignoring the truth, or worse, are they complicit in this masquerade?" DeCola's grievances echo through the void of misunderstanding that surrounds him. His experiences, so vivid and incontrovertible to him, are diminished and dismissed as figments of a troubled mind.

The reduction of his lived reality to mere delusions is a grievous insult, an invalidation that stings with every casual wave of the hand or skeptical glance. DeCola's outcry is not just for acknowledgment but for a fundamental recognition of his humanity, a plea for the community to open their eyes, not just to the dangers he perceives, but to the profound distress of a soul grappling with unseen forces. In his emotional appeals, DeCola seeks not only understanding but a shared sense of urgency, a collective awakening to the shadows he battles alone.

DeCola finds himself wobbling on a precarious edge, where the profound anguish and confusion wrought by his mental state propel him towards thoughts of self-harm and the doom of suicide.

The weight of his suffering makes the idea of escape through such means increasingly enticing. Yet, there exists within him a deep-seated moral and philosophical conflict that serves as a counterbalance to these dark impulses.

At the heart of his hesitation is the ethical quandary that equates the act of taking one's own life with that of committing murder. This internal moral compass, despite being disoriented by his mental turmoil, still points to the inviolable sanctity of life. This principle, deeply ingrained, suggests that life is not just precious but sacred, a notion that introduces a significant pause in his contemplation of suicide.

DeCola's skepticism about the divine does not completely close the door to the possibility of a higher power or a sovereign creator responsible for the gift of life. This sliver of doubt about the absolute absence of a deity introduces a scenario that DeCola finds daunting: the prospect of an afterlife where this creator might confront him. The idea of facing such an entity, having to justify the termination of a life that he did not bring into existence, is a sobering thought. It raises the specter of accountability for negating the very purpose for which his life was presumably intended.

This potential posthumous reckoning suggests not only a violation of a divine plan but also an act of deliberate disrespect towards the ultimate authority, should it exist. The fear that suicide could be seen as a flagrant act of contempt towards this sovereign being plants seeds of doubt in DeCola's mind about the justification of such a decision.

In grappling with these complex ethical, moral, and spiritual dilemmas, DeCola begins to reconsider suicide not as a solution but as a potential worsening of his plight, with far-reaching consequences beyond his current comprehension. This introspection and the consequent acknowledgment of the multifaceted implications of ending one's life led him to a critical juncture where the permanence of suicide thoughts clashes with the evolving nature of his understanding and beliefs. The realization that this act could irreversibly contradict the intentions of a higher power, real or imagined, casts a new light on his predicament, nudging him towards reconsideration and the search for alternative paths through his suffering.

Yet still, DeCola's perception that the world has turned into an adversary, with every element seemingly conspiring against him, intensifies his sense of isolation and despair. His steadfast adherence to an unwavering stance has inadvertently barred the way to any form of betterment, whether it be in his psychological state, physical health, social interactions, or even basic nutritional needs.

DeCola faced a profound dilemma in his community when it came to seeking professional support for his mental health struggles. The resources were not just scarce, but those available fell short of the confidentiality and expertise DeCola desperately sought. This lack of discreet and specialized assistance was a glaring issue, magnified by the prevailing cultural attitudes towards mental health within his community. The prevalent view that mental health issues were a sign of weakness or a spiritual failing left DeCola cornered, unable to voice his battles without fear of judgment.

At the core of DeCola's predicament was his fight with vulnerability. To seek help meant to lay bare his most guarded weaknesses in a communal setting that prized strength and normalcy above all. This internal conflict, the tug-of-war between needing support and the terror of exposing his fragile self, underscored the complexities of DeCola's crisis. His struggle to trust those around him with his mental health woes highlighted the intricate dance between personal vulnerabilities and the broader community dynamics.

Adding another layer to his challenges was DeCola's resistance to incorporating medication into his treatment plan. His apprehension was multi-faceted, with the fear of adverse side effects at the forefront. The thought of these side effects meddling with his daily life or altering his perception was daunting. Moreover, the specter of dependency loomed large, echoing past battles with substance abuse and fueling his reluctance toward medication. This was compounded by the societal stigma surrounding psychiatric medications, painting them as a crutch for the weak. This stigma, perhaps echoed by those closest to him, made the prospect of medication not just a personal crossroads but a societal statement, further entangling DeCola in a web of fear, resistance, and the deep-seated desire for healing.

DeCola harbored profound doubts about the path of medication for his mental health issues. He often found himself questioning the potential benefits, pondering, "Will this really make a difference for me?" or fearing it might only serve as a fleeting fix. These uncertainties were amplified by tales of individuals who didn't find solace in medication, overshadowing the narratives of those who did experience significant improvements.

His inclination leaned heavily towards non-pharmaceutical interventions for managing his mental health, such as engaging in social-oriented therapies, making lifestyle adjustments, or exploring alternative treatments. This preference was deeply rooted in DeCola's values and experiences, as well as a conviction in the efficacy of these methods over traditional medication.

For DeCola, the contemplation of starting medication was entangled with the fear of an altered identity or a loss of emotional control. The idea that medication could potentially dull his emotions or suppress his true self presented a formidable obstacle to accepting medication as part of his treatment plan.

Compounding these concerns was DeCola's skepticism towards the medical establishment. Past encounters that left him feeling misunderstood or sidelined, coupled with a perception that decisions were being hastened, fueled a resistance to adhere to medical recommendations, including the prospect of medication.

DeCola's reluctance to embrace medication underlines the critical need for a patient-centered approach in healthcare. It highlights the importance of healthcare professionals engaging in transparent, empathetic dialogues with their patients. By thoroughly addressing concerns, setting clear expectations, and weighing the benefits against the drawbacks of medication, healthcare providers can ensure that any decision made is well-informed, respecting the patient's autonomy and personal values.

DeCola's Quest for Hope

After his mental breakdown, DeCola's journey morphed into a relentless quest for hope, a quest to navigate through the dimmed corners of his existence confidently. Where life once flowed with the vibrant hues of possibility, he now found himself crossing a grayscale world, each day, a challenge to find even a flicker of light.

Hope, for DeCola, became a scarce commodity, as elusive as a mirage in the desert of his disillusionment. His aspirations and dreams, once clear and within reach, seemed to dissolve into the fog of his present reality. The breakdown not just fractured his mind; it had shattered the lens through which he viewed his future, leaving him to piece together the fragments in search of a picture that held some promise.

Professionally, DeCola grappled with the daunting task of rebuilding a career that mental illness had derailed. The workplace, once a stage for his ambitions, now felt like an arena, each day a battle to prove his worth while wrestling with the internal demons of doubt and inadequacy. The hope for success and fulfillment in his career seemed a distant dream, obscured by the immediate need to stay afloat simply.

Even within the sanctuary of self, hope was a struggle. DeCola fought to reclaim the fragments of his identity scattered by the storm of his breakdown. Self-doubt lurked in the shadows of his mind, whispering insidious comparisons between his current self and the person he used to be. The journey back to self-acceptance, to viewing his reflection and recognizing the person staring back, was fraught with setbacks and self-recrimination.

During DeCola's mental health crisis, hope was a beacon that flickered in the darkness, its light waxing and waning with the tides of his inner turmoil. For DeCola, hope was not a constant; it was a delicate, transient entity that danced on the edges of his consciousness, appearing in those rare moments of tranquility or when he felt the comforting presence of those who stood by him. Yet, this hope was often eclipsed by the formidable shadows of doubt and despair that clouded his vision, making the journey toward optimism a tumultuous voyage through stormy seas.

The scaffolding of DeCola's hope was significantly influenced by the strength and presence of his support network. Words of encouragement and acts of kindness from friends, family, and dedicated mental health professionals acted as pillars that upheld his fragile sense of hope, illuminating the possibility of a brighter tomorrow. In contrast, a void in this support network could magnify his feelings of isolation, causing the light of hope to dim and recede into the recesses of his mind, making the path forward seem daunting and lonely.

DeCola's inner fortitude and the strategies he employed to navigate his emotional landscape played pivotal roles in his dance with hope. Moments of resilience—be it through introspection, therapeutic revelations, or the solace found in hobbies and passions—were like sparks in the darkness, re-igniting the flame of hope within him. However, when these coping mechanisms faltered or seemed inadequate, hope became a distant, flickering star in the vast night sky of his struggles.

The societal lens through which mental health is viewed, alongside personal and professional pressures and the broader context of global events, also cast their shadows on DeCola's sense of hope. When the world seemed to shift in a positive direction, hope's glow grew warmer, but adverse changes could just as quickly cast it back into a cool shadow. The unpredictable nature of his mental health journey the ambiguity surrounding potential treatments, and their outcomes added a heavy cloak of uncertainty, making hope a difficult sentiment to grasp and hold onto.

Yet, amidst the disruption of his ordeal, DeCola occasionally found beacons of clarity and insight—rare, precious moments that cut through the fog of despair. These realizations about his inherent strengths, the transient nature of his current state, and the inherent potential for transformation acted as lighthouses guiding him back to the shores of hope. They reminded him that the dark waters he navigated were not endless, that change was possible, and that a calmer sea might lie ahead.

The journey of recovery, DeCola found, was marked not by grandiose leaps but by the small, steady steps he took each day. Every moment that felt even marginally better than the last was a victory, a sign that hope was not just a distant dream but a potential reality. In navigating the complexities of his mental health crisis, hope became not just a feeling but a journey—a mosaic of highs and lows, each piece reflecting the multifaceted nature of his struggle and resilience. Through this journey, DeCola learned that hope, in its essence, is both a gift and a challenge, an ever-changing companion on the road to healing and recovery.

At the zenith of DeCola's mental health crisis, his aspirations for academic achievement and professional success were entangled in a complex web of personal and societal challenges, reflecting the profound impact such crises can exert on an individual's life goals and direction. This confluence of factors—ranging from internal self-doubts to external societal pressures—painted a daunting landscape for DeCola, making the journey toward education or employment seem not just challenging but, at times, impossible.

The relentless tide of mental health struggles washed away much of DeCola's self-confidence and belief in his capabilities, casting long shadows over his aspirations. The once-clear path to academic success or career advancement became obscured as his inner voice of doubt questioned his adequacy and ability to thrive in such demanding environments. This erosion of self-belief left DeCola standing at a crossroads, with the path ahead shrouded in fog.

Fear became a constant companion for DeCola—fear of not measuring up to the rigors of coursework, fear of faltering in a professional setting, and the chilling prospect of rejection. This fear was not just about failing to meet external benchmarks but was deeply tied to the potential of his mental health struggles coming to light, adding another layer of vulnerability in his pursuit of education or employment.

DeCola's mental health crisis cast a long shadow over his perceptive faculties, making concentration, memory retention, and motivation scarce commodities. Tasks that once seemed straightforward now loomed as Herculean challenges, further feeding his cycle of doubt and hesitation about his academic and professional capabilities.

The societal stigma surrounding mental health erected invisible barriers around DeCola, adding weight to his decision-making process. The dilemma of disclosing his mental health status to educational institutions or prospective employers was fraught with concerns about potential bias, misunderstanding, or outright discrimination, further complicating his path forward.

Amidst this turmoil, the future appeared not as a horizon of endless possibilities but as a network of uncertainty. This uncertainty made the act of planning for the future, of committing to the pursuit of education or a career, a task riddled with anxiety and indecision, casting gloom over DeCola's once-bright aspirations.

Financial concerns, too, intertwined with DeCola's mental health struggles, adding a tangible strain to his aspirations. The financial implications of pursuing further education or the need for stable employment became daunting considerations, entwined with the costs of managing his mental health and the potential impact on his ability to work.

The isolating nature of DeCola's mental health crisis may have severed ties with peers and potential support networks, which are often lifelines in navigating the complexities of academic and professional endeavors. This isolation not only magnified the challenges he faced but also diminished the sources of hope and encouragement that are vital in such journeys.

DeCola's story, marked by the intersection of mental health challenges with personal and professional aspirations, underscores the resilience and courage required to navigate such turbulent waters. It highlights the need for a comprehensive support system that addresses not only the mental health aspects but also provides academic and career guidance, fostering a community where hope can flourish and perseverance is celebrated.

During the peak of his mental health crisis, DeCola found himself entangled in a profound struggle with the concept of hope and the prospect of a brighter tomorrow. This struggle was not just about battling his current predicaments but also about confronting the daunting specter of the future, making it an intensely personal and multifaceted ordeal.

The overwhelming nature of his present circumstances cast a long shadow over DeCola's ability to look beyond the immediate horizon. Each day's trials and tribulations consumed his thoughts and energy, rendering the future a distant, murky concept rather than a beacon of potential and opportunity. The very notion of 'tomorrow' seemed disconnected from his reality, as if the future was a foreign land beyond his reach, where hope might reside but felt inaccessible amidst his current turmoil.

The unpredictability and vulnerability inherent in DeCola's mental health crisis amplified his apprehensions about the unknown facets of the future. This fear of what lay ahead was not just about facing new challenges but also about the potential continuation or intensification of his current struggles. The inability to predict or control the trajectory of his mental health added layers of anxiety and trepidation to his thoughts about what tomorrow might bring, especially when today was already fraught with difficulties.

Past experiences with mental health challenges, replete with their disappointments and setbacks, cast a long, ominous shadow over DeCola's outlook on the future. These memories acted as constant reminders of his vulnerabilities, making the prospect of overcoming current obstacles and achieving a semblance of hope for the future seem like a challenging task. The fear that history might repeat itself, that the patterns of despair and struggle would continue unabated, tainted his ability to envisage a hopeful tomorrow.

Isolation compounded DeCola's sense of despair regarding the future. The feeling of being adrift disconnected from the support and understanding of others, can profoundly impact one's ability to foster hope. Human connections, which often serve as lifelines in times of crisis, seemed frayed or non-existent for DeCola, making the future appear even more desolate and foreboding.

The stigma and misconceptions surrounding mental health posed additional barriers to DeCola's sense of hope. Encounters with judgment, misunderstanding, or outright dismissal of his struggles could have deepened his sense of alienation, making the idea of a brighter future seem not just improbable but unworthy of pursuit. The societal stigma attached to mental health can magnify feelings of shame and diminish one's belief in the possibility of positive change.

In the midst of a profound mental health crisis, DeCola embarked on a journey marked by existential turmoil and a quest for meaning. The future, obscured by the dense fog of uncertainty, seemed empty of both purpose and promise, casting a shadow over his aspirations for a brighter tomorrow. Yet, it was within this very struggle that the seeds of hope began to sprout, nurtured by small yet significant victories that emerged as beacons in the darkness.

These moments, though modest in isolation, collectively forged a path toward incremental healing. The warmth of a friend's smile, the completion of a simple task, or a fleeting instance of self-forgiveness each served as a testament to DeCola's resilience. They illuminated the possibility of a future where hope was not just an elusive dream but a tangible reality within grasp.

As DeCola navigated the turbulent waters of his crisis, each victory, no matter how slight, reaffirmed the potential for joy and fulfillment amidst adversity. These glimmers of light, found in everyday achievements and connections, gradually wove hope into the fabric of his daily life. It was a gentle yet persistent force, guiding him towards a future where the dark clouds of despair began to part, revealing a horizon imbued with the promise of brighter days.

This journey underscored the critical importance of compassionate support and understanding in overcoming life's trials. It highlighted the undeniable strength found in hope, a quiet yet powerful beacon that guides us back to light, step by cautious step, even in the darkest of times.

DeCola yearned for a kind of breakthrough that would not only recognize but fully embrace the complexities of his challenges. He envisioned a solution emerging from self-reliance or the compassionate understanding of his family and friends. He hoped they could truly grasp the multifaceted nature of his ordeal, which intertwined psychological upheavals with possible physical implications.

His reflections on possible routes to navigate through his inner turmoil highlighted paths that offered more than mere treatment. He sought a profound comprehension and management of his condition, aspiring for solutions that transcended conventional remedies. He occasionally contemplated the role of mental health experts, with their intricate understanding of the human psyche and arsenal of therapeutic techniques as a possibility as they held out the promise of not just easing his present distress but also guiding him on a transformative journey toward healing and insight. They offered a semblance of order in the midst of his chaos, a chance to recapture the bright horizons of tomorrow that seemed so distant amid his darkest moments. Yet, for an extended period, DeCola had retreated into the sanctuary of his mind, convinced of his ability to confront the storms of his condition single-handedly. The idea of seeking external support initially seemed at odds with his cherished self-reliance, feeling almost like an intrusion on his deeply valued autonomy.

Chapter 3: The Realization

During DeCola's relentless emotional storm, a moment of profound clarity emerged, as delicate and fleeting as a solitary raindrop caressing a parched leaf under the protective embrace of ancient trees. This brief instant bore the heavy silence of countless unspoken words and a surge of emotions long ignored. Amidst an activity as unremarkable as browsing through old photographs on an afternoon bathed in gentle sunlight, DeCola's world shifted subtly yet irrevocably.

Each photograph, a frozen echo of joyous past moments, seemed to whisper of a life brimming with color and vitality, a sharp and painful contrast to the dull, ominous existence that now gripped DeCola. The once vibrant memories, now just pictorial images, slipped through his shaking hands, each one a reminder of what had been and what now seemed an impossible distance away.

As the photos fluttered to the floor, like leaves in an autumn breeze, they stirred something jerky within DeCola. It was as if each image, each captured laugh and shared smiley posture, shook the fragile layers enclosing his bottled-up emotions. And then, as inevitably as a dam yielding to the relentless pressure of the waters it has been holding back, DeCola's defenses crumbled.

The floodgates opened, releasing a deluge of pent-up fears, swirling doubts, and the profound ache of tears that had been staunchly repressed. This moment, unremarkable in its setting but notable in its impact on DeCola, marked a pivotal chapter in his journey through the storm of his crisis. It was a stark reminder of the depth of his emotional turmoil, a call to acknowledge and confront the tangled web of feelings he had endeavored to navigate alone.

DeCola's journey through his turmoil was akin to navigating an intricate, shadowy maze, with each turn and twist leading him further into an abyss of despair. Alone, without the compass of professional therapy or the anchor of medical support, he found himself lost in a vast expanse of confusion and sorrow. This lack of a structured, nurturing framework for his care meant that he was effectively in a state of limbo, unable to move forward or find a way out of his mental entanglement. The absence of these guiding lights in his life not only deepened his sense of isolation but also magnified the emotional and psychological strain he bore each day.

As he ventured deeper into this metaphorical labyrinth, the isolation became more pronounced, enveloping him in a silence that echoed the void of external support. This isolation wasn't just physical but deeply psychological, creating barriers that seemed impossible. The absence of a guiding hand to lead him through the complexities of his condition meant that every effort to break free from this cycle of despair was met with the unyielding walls of his own mind's making.

The toll this journey took on DeCola was profound. The constant battle against his thoughts and feelings, without any form of relief or external intervention, led to an ever-increasing burden. Hope, once a distant but visible beacon in his life, began to fade, its light dimming to the faintest of glows. With each day that passed in this state of standstill, the possibility of finding a way out of the darkness seemed to recede further into the distance.

This relentless cycle of solitude and stagnation created a feedback loop of despair, where the absence of professional care not only hindered his progress but actively contributed to the deepening of his predicament. The very essence of hope, which thrives on the prospect of change and improvement, was eroded by the constancy of his unchanging circumstances, leaving DeCola to grapple with the shadows of what could have been if only he had reached out for the help that lay just beyond the confines of his self-imposed solitude.

It wasn't until DeCola found himself at a critical juncture, a precipice where the pain of remaining the same outweighed the fear of change, that he experienced a seismic shift in perspective. Confronted with the stark reality of his condition and the profound sense of loss for the time and opportunities squandered in his steadfast resistance, DeCola reached an inflection point. This moment of stark realization, a profound reckoning with the depths of his despair, catalyzed a transformative decision.

Reluctantly, yet with a burgeoning sense of necessity, DeCola reconsidered the very support he had long declined. It was a decision fraught with vulnerability and the painful acknowledgment of his limitations. In this act of conceding to seek professional help, DeCola embarked on a new chapter. It was a journey towards healing, marked by the tentative embrace of therapeutic guidance, the potential of medical intervention, and the foundational support of proper nutrition.

This pivotal decision, born from a moment of profound personal crisis, marked the beginning of DeCola's slow but steadfast journey out of the shadows of despair and into the light of recovery and renewal.

It wasn't until DeCola reached the pivotal moment, a critical crossroads where the agony of maintaining the status quo surpassed his fear of change, that a significant transformation began to take shape. Faced with the harsh truth of his situation and the profound realization of the time and opportunities lost to his unwavering resistance, he arrived at the turning point. This moment of clarity, this deep confrontation with his despair, sparked a crucial change in perspective.

The choice to consider professional help was born from a place of empowerment, an act of informed decision-making rather than a move of last resort. DeCola recognized that each decision he made—each nod of consent—wove a distinct pattern into the fabric of his mental health journey. The acknowledgment that his staunch dedication to self-determination has apparently extended his suffering marked a significant shift in perspective.

Viewing professional intervention through this new lens, DeCola reframed it as an opportunity for growth and healing, a pathway he could choose to walk down, not one forced upon him. This evolution in his mindset, rooted in a deep respect for his agency, promised to transform the terrain of his mental health journey from one marked by solitude to one illuminated by the prospects of collaborative recovery.

This newfound resolve was met with a mixture of excitement and caution from DeCola's family. Aware of his right to retract his consent at any point, they navigated this delicate phase with a blend of urgency and restraint. Their actions were guided by an understanding of the critical nature of this moment, yet they were careful not to exert undue pressure, mindful of DeCola's longstanding quest for autonomy.

The family sprang into action, meticulously researching and consulting with esteemed mental health organizations and specialists. Their efforts were centered around DeCola, ensuring that every piece of information gathered and every decision made was done with his active involvement and consent. The selection of any mental health professional was left entirely to DeCola, underscoring his leading role in his healing process. He was also given the autonomy to decide if and which family member he wished to have by his side during consultations, further emphasizing his control over his journey.

As plans solidified and appointments scheduled, the family's commitment to supporting DeCola was palpable. Their readiness to adapt their schedules and make necessary adjustments reflected the collective resolve to confront and navigate this challenging period together. This concerted effort, driven by love and respect for DeCola's autonomy, heralded a hopeful chapter, one that promised not just the possibility of recovery but a deeper understanding and connection within the family, united in their commitment to DeCola's wellbeing.

The realization was as sharp as it was profound; the struggles DeCola had been dismissing as mere ripples were, in fact, the tides of a looming storm if not promptly addressed. The veneer of resilience, worn so proudly, began to crack, revealing the depth of the crisis that lay beneath. It was no longer a matter of simply soldiering on; it was a clarion call for help, a beacon lit in the darkness of denial.

In a pivotal moment of self-realization and increasing hope, DeCola made the decisive step to fully integrate professional support in confronting his mental health challenges. A crucial part of this journey involved capturing the essence of his tumultuous experience in his own words, untainted and uninterrupted. He proposed a unique approach: to have his story documented verbatim by a neutral party, someone detached from the emotional complexities of his family dynamic. This request was not just about preserving his narrative but about anchoring his reality in preparation for the therapeutic journey ahead.

DeCola's insistence on an impartial listener underscored his desire for authenticity and objectivity, traits he valued deeply, even during his crisis. He believed that a comprehensive and unaltered account of his experiences would provide a solid foundation for his interactions with mental health professionals. This narrative, he reasoned, would not only aid his memory but also offer the therapists a clear, undiluted insight into his world, facilitating a more targeted and effective intervention.

DeCola's approach to sharing his personal story with mental health professionals is both innovative and deeply insightful. By requesting that each professional listen to a recorded version of his story before meeting him, DeCola emphasizes the importance of understanding the patient's journey in its entirety. This method ensures that each professional is fully acquainted with his experiences, challenges, and perspectives, fostering a more personalized and effective consultation.

The significance of this approach lies in its potential to save precious time during face-to-face consultations, allowing for a deeper dive into the most pertinent issues without the need for repetitive storytelling. This method respects the time of both the patient and the professionals, optimizing their interactions for maximum benefit.

Moreover, DeCola's insistence on the return of each recording after it has been listened to, coupled with the emphasis on confidentiality and data protection, showcases his awareness and concern for privacy and ethical treatment. This not only protects his narrative but also sets a standard for how sensitive information should be handled within the mental health care system.

DeCola's story and his method of sharing it highlight the importance of patient-centered care, where understanding and respecting the patient's narrative is pivotal. It serves as a call to action for mental health professionals to prioritize listening and understanding as foundational aspects of care. This innovative approach could inspire changes in how patient histories are gathered and utilized, leading to more compassionate, efficient, and effective mental health care practices.

The family, recognizing the significance of DeCola's request and the shift in his attitude towards seeking help, quickly concurred. Arrangements were made to bring in a media professional who could capture DeCola's account with the fidelity and neutrality it demanded. This step was more than just a practical preparation for therapy; it was a symbolic act of taking control, a testament to DeCola's readiness to confront and work through the complexities of his condition.

As DeCola narrated his story, he delved into the depths of his experiences, recounting the intricacies of his perceived reality with a clarity and coherence that bellied the turmoil within. This recorded narrative, set against the backdrop of his long-standing resistance to external intervention, marked a significant milestone in his journey. It was an act of vulnerability, of trust in the process, and ultimately, a tangible manifestation of his hope that change was possible.

This initial step of documenting his story was not just about setting a reference for future therapy sessions; it was an emotional outburst exercise for DeCola, a chance to externalize his inner turmoil and see his experiences from a new perspective. It was a bridge between the isolation of his mental struggles and the collaborative path of recovery that lies ahead. With this recorded narrative, DeCola not only preserved his memories but also laid down the first stone on his path to healing, signaling a readiness to explore the depths of his psyche with the guidance of professionals, bolstered by the renewed hope of reclaiming his life from the shadows of his mind.

DeCola's Quest for Understanding

As DeCola's inclination shifted towards receiving professional support, he understandably embarked on a relevant quest for understanding in a world that suddenly seemed written in a foreign script. Conversations turned into mazes, where words twisted and turned, eluding his grasp. The straightforward dialogue he once navigated with ease now felt like riddles wrapped in enigmas, leaving him perpetually on the outside, gazing in.

His interactions became exercises in frustration as if he were tuning into a radio frequency just out of range, catching snippets of clarity amidst a sea of static. The more he strained to understand, the more elusive comprehension became. Friends and family, their intentions no doubt genuine, seemed to speak in a dialect of concern that DeCola couldn't decode. Their attempts to connect, to offer solace or advice, often missed the mark, landing in spaces filled with misinterpretations and misunderstandings.

In his professional life, the breakdown had erected barriers where there were none, turning collaborative efforts into solo ventures through unfamiliar territory. Instructions that once made perfect sense now seemed coded; tasks that should have been straightforward morphed into complex puzzles that DeCola couldn't piece together.

Even within the confines of his mind, understanding proved elusive. His thoughts, once coherent and linear, now danced to an erratic rhythm, dodging his attempts to corral them into order. Emotions surged without warning, defying his efforts to understand their origins or stem their tide. The internal dialogue that had guided him through life's challenges became a cacophony of conflicting voices, each clamoring for attention yet offering no clarity.

In this landscape of confusion, DeCola's quest for understanding was less about seeking answers from the external world and more about learning to navigate the tumultuous waters of his inner realm. The challenge was no longer about making sense of others' words and actions but about deciphering the language of his psyche, understanding the whispers of his heart amidst the clamor of his mind.

This journey toward understanding was a path marked by introspection and self-discovery, a process of peeling back the layers to reveal the raw, unvarnished truth of his experience. It was a pilgrimage to the core of his being, where the seeds of comprehension lay buried beneath the debris of his breakdown. In this quest, each glimmer of insight, no matter how fleeting, was a beacon, illuminating the way forward through the fog of confusion that shrouded his world.

Along the journey through a notable and timely in-depth reflection, DeCola recapitulated that his mental health was

fundamentally ignited by a profoundly disturbing and disorienting traumatic experience, the origins of which are
shrouded in ambiguity and fear. According to DeCola, the
onset of his crisis was marked by an encounter that defies
easy explanation or categorization within the realms of conventional reality.

DeCola found himself at an intersection of reality and
imagination, struggling to distinguish whether his recounted
tale was woven from the threads of dreams, visions, and
trances or if it was intertwined with tangible daily encounters. Yet, despite this ambiguity, the profound impact of his
experiences was undeniable, leaving an indelible mark on
every aspect of his existence. The sheer intensity of the
events he described transcended the need for clarification,
painting a vivid interlacing of influence that adorned the entirety of his crisis.

He recounts being overwhelmed by a group of six enigmatic figures whose presence and conduct were unlike anything familiar or human. These beings, described as towering and fearsome, seemed to transcend the ordinary, bearing
more resemblance to creatures of myth or cinema than to
flesh-and-blood individuals. Their appearance was notable
for its otherworldliness, with bodies clad in what appeared

to be bronze armor, exuding an aura of invincibility and cold detachment.

The interaction with these figures was characterized by a profound sense of helplessness and violation, as DeCola describes being treated with a mercilessness that stripped away any semblance of dignity or humanity. The beings' intent was clear and unyielding, their actions geared towards the fulfillment of a mysterious mission, the nature of which remained obscure to DeCola. His resistance was met with force, and his plea for help went unanswered, deepening the sense of isolation and terror that enveloped the experience.

An act of physical violation marked the climax of this harrowing episode— an injection followed by surgery process which seemingly led to the embedding of a digital chip in his brain that led to a loss of consciousness, leaving De-Cola to grapple with the terrifying possibility that he might not wake up again! The subsequent return to consciousness, devoid of the presence of these beings, offered no solace or clarity, only a lingering sense of having been irrevocably changed by the encounter.

This earliest experience, igniting the re of the crisis, re-counted DeCola, plunged him into the depths of psychological trauma, where the lines between reality and delusion blur. The vividness of the experience, coupled with the inability to anchor it within the familiar, laid the groundwork for a mental health crisis rooted in the struggle to make sense of the incomprehensible. The aftermath of this encounter left DeCola in a state of perpetual unrest, haunted by the shadows of beings whose existence de es rational explanation, yet whose impact on his soul is indelibly real.

DeCola's narrative takes a darker turn as he recounts the aftermath of his harrowing encounter with the six enigmatic figures. Emerging from the ordeal with a pounding migraine that seemed to localize in one side of his head, DeCola experienced an unexpected fundamental shift in his reality. From the deadly experience of the intense pain, a familiar voice breaks the silence, markedly different from the menacing brutality of his initial captors. This voice, soft and soothing, offered a stark contrast to the unkind treatment DeCola had just endured, its melodic rhymes providing a semblance of comfort in the wake of his trauma. Nonetheless, DeCola later realized he was sincerely mistaken.

As the seemingly benevolent voice played games with his mind, referring to the operation that had just taken place, it hints at an extraordinary transformation that had supposedly elevated DeCola to a superhuman status. DeCola contemplated the recent encounter might be the actualization of the poetic promises earlier made to him at the onset of his trials. The notion that he had not only survived but emerged stronger from the nightmare was both perplexing and strangely reassuring. The voice, with its poetic timbre, seemed to weave a narrative of empowerment and belonging, welcoming DeCola into the ranks of the 'elites'—a supposed cadre of individuals who wielded significant influence over the world. Poetically, the voice re-echoed the spurious supernatural experience:

"Veiled in ignorance, your vision clears,

Beyond the tongue, your tastebuds enjoy.

Softest murmurs, your ears they steer,

Past floral bloom scents draw you near.

Through invisible layers, your senses adhere."

This narrative, as fantastical as it sounded, offered De-Cola a sense of purpose and identity in the immediate aftermath of his trauma. The voice's assurance that his harrowing experience was an initiation, a rite of passage into a realm of heightened intellect and influence, provided a framework through which to interpret his suffering. It suggested that the pain and terror were not in vain but were instead the price of admission to a transformative yet mysterious new existence.

Despite the allure of this newfound 'membership' and the soothing quality of the voice, DeCola's intuitive anger at the violation of his autonomy lingered. The voice's attempt to rationalize the trauma as a necessary step towards greatness did little to quell the surge of resentment he felt at being coerced into this torment. Yet, his physical condition— marked by severe headaches— muted his capacity to protest or seek clarity, trapping him in a silent struggle with his thoughts and the bewildering narrative unfolding within his mind.

This continuation of DeCola's story reveals a complex interplay of physical pain, psychological trauma, and the desperate search for meaning in the face of an inexplicable and life-altering event. The introduction of the benevolent voice serves as a coping mechanism, offering a narrative of empowerment to counterbalance the terror of his abduction and the lingering effects of his ordeal. Yet, beneath the surface of this apparent induction into a higher ranking of existence, DeCola wrestles with the fundamental violation of his will and the profound implications of his imposed transformation.

DeCola's affinity for poetry and music, passions that had long provided solace and joy, became the very channels through which the obscure voice snared his attention, even amidst the snag of unbearable pain. The voice, with its melodic cadence and poetic allure, spoke of an awakening, a transformation that promised to elevate DeCola's sensory experiences to a realm beyond the ordinary.

To DeCola, the message of the bodyless voice was clear: his perception of the world was about to transcend the limitations of the mundane. His eyes, once bound to the tangible, would now pierce through the veil of the physical to behold sights reserved for a chosen few. The voice assured him that his taste would be enhanced, enabling him to discern flavors with a precision that surpassed the capabilities of an ordinary palate, hinting at a deeper, perhaps symbolic, ingestion of experiences.

His ears, the voice whispered, would become attuned to the supernatural conversations of unseen entities, granting him direct access to a symphony of whispers that eluded mortal hearing. This promise of auditory transcendence suggested a communion with voices that existed just beyond the limitations of the known.

The voice spoke of an olfactory awakening, where DeCola's sense of smell would be heightened to detect the sublime fragrances of realms unseen, scents that carried the essence of otherworldliness. This sensory expansion hinted at a connection to a world that was perceptible as well as elusive, one that ordinary beings could scarcely imagine.

And perhaps, most compelling was the promise that DeCola's entire being would become sensitive to the extraordinary caress of invisible forces. The voice enticed him with the prospect of feeling the intangible, of being touched by hands, not of this world, suggesting an intimate fondling with the paranormal.

At that moment, the voice, with its poetic delivery and tempting promises, tapped into DeCola's deepest yearnings for understanding and transcending desires. It lured him into a world permeated with strange and extraordinary experiences, where the boundaries of reality were not just expanded but obliterated. DeCola, despite the lingering pain and the shadows of doubt, found himself drawn into the seductive embrace of this new, enigmatic existence, captivated by the allure of sensing the world in a way he never thought possible.

DeCola found himself at the crossroads of enchantment and skepticism at the promises unfolded before him, offering a glimpse into a realm beyond the ordinary. The prospect of transcending human limitations and delving into the mysteries that lay hidden from the average mind was undeniably compelling. The allure of becoming something more, of stepping into a role that set him apart from the masses, was a siren call to his ego, promising a status elevated beyond his wildest dreams. He was somewhat oblivious to the trap he had fallen into.

Yet, beneath the covering of these impressive promises, DeCola's rational mind harbored deep-seated apprehensions. The transformation into a being capable of perceiving the unfathomable depths of the universe was not without its daunting implications. He was acutely aware of his humanity, with all its inherent frailties and bounds. The thought of being thrust into the vast, strange expanse of an "endless universe" stirred a primal fear within him. How would he, a creature of earth and flesh, navigate the overwhelming infinity that lay beyond the familiar confines of his planet? The enormity of such an existence, with its unknown variables and potential perils, loomed large, casting a shadow of doubt over the seductive narrative fashioned by the hidden voice.

DeCola's skepticism was further fueled by the anonymity of his enigmatic guide. The absence of a physical presence of the seemingly harmless tone and the reluctance to reveal a face or form is equally an unsettling encounter, perhaps more mind-boggling than the visible bronze-armored beings. This invisibility raised questions in DeCola's mind regarding the credibility and intentions of the voice. If the promises held, if the path to superhuman capabilities was genuine, why then is the instructor behind the voice remaining hidden since DeCola had gained spiritual status?

The legitimate concerns highlighted the chasm between the allure of transcendent abilities and the reality of DeCola's human condition. The duality of his desire for extraordinary experiences and his innate caution in the face of the unknown painted a complex portrait of a puzzled young man on the brink of a transformative journey, one nervous with the potential for both unparalleled discovery and unforeseen consequences.

DeCola's conviction that he had transcended the bounds of ordinary human existence was deeply rooted in the transformative aftermath of his harrowing encounter. The ordeal, marked by its intensity and the inexplicable nature of the events he experienced, catalyzed a profound shift in his self-perception. This shift was not merely an adjustment but a complete overhaul of his understanding of reality and his place within it.

The sense of being superhuman emerged from the stark contrast between his newfound perceptions and the seemingly mundane understanding of those around him. DeCola interpreted others' perception of him and his misconception of others as a testament to his elevated status. In his mind, the inability of people to grasp his reality was not a reaction to his altered state but a confirmation of their limited awareness. He saw himself as privy to a dimension of existence that remained veiled to the average person as he was endowed with insights and powers that set him apart.

This belief was further reinforced by the directives issued by the enigmatic controller, who guided DeCola into the realms and experiences that defied his prior understanding of the world. The journey into this "strange world," as DeCola described it, was not just a physical or metaphysical voyage but a symbolic induction into a select group of individuals, human and yet "superhuman". The notion of being "specially chosen" for this journey imbued DeCola with a sense of exclusivity and privilege, intensifying his belief in his extraordinary nature.

The chip-controller's instructions, which DeCola felt compelled to follow, represent the new navigation tool to this newfound identity, each directive serving to further distance him from his former self and deeper into the embrace of his perceived superhuman capabilities. The narrative of being one of the "few candidates" for this "uncommon adventure" not only elevated DeCola's sense of self but also created a dichotomy between him and the rest of humanity. In this dichotomous worldview, DeCola saw himself as part of an elite, transcendent minority endowed with powers and insights beyond the reach of ordinary mortals.

Thus, the foundation of DeCola's deluded belief in his superhuman status was a complex interplay of his altered perceptions, the validation from an unseen guide, and the stark contrast between his experiences and the understanding of those around him. This confluence of factors created a self-reinforcing cycle, where each element validated and amplified the others, cementing DeCola's conviction in his extraordinary transformation.

DeCola was briefed on the extraordinary voyage. His mind is imbued with a guide to navigate the enigmatic realm that lies ahead. He learned that while he would not journey alone, the peculiar nature of this expedition meant that fellow travelers would remain invisible to one another. Each participant was assured a singular interactive experience within the mysterious domain, the uniqueness of which is shaped by each distinct participating personality and the powers bestowed.

Despite an undercurrent of trepidation about the venture, DeCola felt cornered into participation. He had been starkly cautioned about the dire consequences of defying the directives of the chip-embedded controller. The most harrowing retribution threat for the non-compliant was a perpetual torment for the already transformed nature by an unseen, scorching force. The warning also extended to a prohibition against sharing the experiences of foreign beings with any human, as the omnipresent chip monitors every move.

DeCola, in a wordless wish, expressed a desperate plea for rescue from the eternal anguish that loomed over him. Guided by the shadowy entity, his journey unfolded through a labyrinth of aerial maneuvers, where he found himself adrift, soaring and hovering with the whims of an unseen force. The journey's pace fluctuated unpredictably, at times passive and hovering at others, hurtling forward with the velocity of a rocket. DeCola was but a passenger, bereft of control over his trajectory or speed, surrendered to the absolute dominion of the controlling entity. The duration of this surreal voyage remained an enigma, lost in the timeless expanse of his extraordinary adventure.

Upon reaching the border's enigmatic destination, DeCola found himself on the fringes of a forest that defied all logic and reason, a place where darkness should have reigned supreme were it not for the luminous flora casting an ethereal glow upon the woodland floor. This natural light show rendered everything in vivid detail, from the minuscule ants embarking on their ground-level expeditions to their tree-scaling counterparts navigating the bark highways.

Yet, amidst this illuminated wonderland, it wasn't the radiant underbrush that seized DeCola's fascination but the forest's eccentric inhabitants. The array of animals and beings that called this place home was as bewildering as it was hilarious. The monkeys stole the show with their ludicrous antics and otherworldly appearances. These weren't your garden-variety primates; they were a riot of evolutionary mishaps and fantastic acrobats.

Among them were headless gymnasts, defying gravity and logic in equal measure, swinging from branch to branch with ease that bellied their lack of cranial navigation. Then there were the multi-headed variants, each head seemingly possessing its distinct personality, leading to comical disputes over which direction to leap next. Limbs seemed to be an optional accessory in this arboreal circus, with some monkeys sporting an excess of arms and legs, turning their tree-top routines into a chaotic flurry of appendages, while others, devoid of tails and limbs, managed to bob and weave through the foliage with the grace of a feather caught in a breeze.

The spectacle was further amplified by the monkeys' apparent obliviousness to the absence of music, their movements synchronized to silent rhythms only they could perceive. Their enthusiastic glances towards DeCola, coupled with animated gestures, seemed like an open invitation to join their silent disco in the treetops. DeCola, however, found himself too tangled in his web of worries to entertain the idea of participating in their headless, multi-limbed jamboree.

In this bizarre display, where nature had seemingly thrown all rules out the window, DeCola stood as the lone spectator to a comedy of the absurd, a performance so weird it bordered on the comical yet so captivating in its oddity that it was impossible to look away.

As the novelty of the monkeys' bizarre antics began to wear thin, DeCola's amusement gave way to a heightened sense of irritation. The relentless gymnastics, once a source of bewildered entertainment, now seemed nothing more than a repetitive circus act devoid of charm. The forest, with its radiant vegetation and headless acrobats, transformed in DeCola's eyes from a place of fantastic wonder to a theatre of the ridiculous, where the line between amusing and annoying was increasingly blurred.

Amid the already chaotic scene of headless acrobatics and multi-limbed dance routines, the monkeys introduced a new, rather unsavory element to their performance. With a lack of decorum that only these forest jesters could muster, they began to defecate and urinate from their lofty perches with reckless abandon. The forest floor, and indeed the air itself, became a veritable mine field of monkey missiles.

DeCola's frustration boiled over as he witnessed the monkeys' antics, which appeared to be nothing short of mockery. Their wide-open mouths, revealing less-than-pleasant dental displays, seemed to him like jeers, their laughter ringing in his ears as a chorus of scorn. The clamor they made, coupled with their hysterical neck gyrations, painted a picture of wild jubilation that DeCola couldn't help but interpret as directed at his expense. This perceived ridicule, a blatant disrespect set against the backdrop of their chaotic excitement, was pushing DeCola to the edge.

DeCola, already at his wit's end with the relentless festivities, now found himself dodging these impromptu aerial assaults. It was as if the monkeys, in their boundless enthusiasm, had decided to add an interactive dimension to their performance, much to DeCola's dismay. The spectacle turned into a bizarre game of dodgeball, except the balls were, well, not decent balls.

With each close call, DeCola's frustration turned into a frantic dance of evasion, his movements becoming as erratic and unpredictable as those of his primate tormentors. Unconsciously, he became a participant in the game he detested. His vigilance reached new heights, his eyes darting skyward, not in awe but in wary anticipation of the next drop. The irony of the situation wasn't lost on him; here he was, supposedly endowed with extraordinary powers, yet his most immediate concern was avoiding being showered by the monkeys' waste.

The absurdity of the situation was more than a joke. It was an interesting reminder. DeCola, the reluctant star of this primate-produced display, narrowly escaped one unsightly splatter after another. His predicament would have been humorous to an outside observer, a man of supposed superhuman status engaged in a desperate ballet to avoid becoming the unwilling canvas for mere monkey artistry. Yet, for DeCola, each successful dodge was a small victory, a testament to his determination not to be dampened, quite literally, by the ruthless ridicule of the tree-clinging co-inhabitants.

As the monkeys' ceaseless celebration continued unabated, DeCola's patience frayed to its breaking point. The spectacle, initially amusing, now seemed a mockery of his predicament. He was torn between two interpretations: either the primates were blatantly disregarding his presence with their antics, or, more unsettlingly, he was simply invisible to them. This ambiguity fueled his frustration, especially as some monkeys, in moments of wild abandon, flashed their colored teeth with mouths tightly closed behind the teeth, with much enthusiasm that DeCola found increasingly intolerable. The sight of their unbridled joy, in stark contrast to his growing agitation, pushed him to a moment of overreaction, where he declared, with fervent exasperation, that he had unequivocally reached his limit.

The incessant performances, the silent music to which these peculiar creatures danced, became a tiresome spectacle that overstretched DeCola's nerves. His initial fascination curdled into exasperation as the realization dawned on him that he was trapped in an endless loop of clownish routines. The desire to return to the familiar comforts of home, to escape this maddening display of unimaginable absurdity, was overwhelming.

In the seemingly reckless demonstration, DeCola stood, torn between the desire to express his frustration and the realization of the futility of such endeavors. The forest, with its illuminated trees and headless jesters, no longer held the attraction of escapism but had become a stage for a performance that had lost its overall brilliance, leaving DeCola yearning for an intervention call that never came.

Caught in this whirlwind of frustration, DeCola let out an involuntary groan, a deep, guttural sound that seemed to echo the depths of his growing despair. It was a moment of unguarded emotional release, a manifestation of the depression that was creeping in, casting a shadow over the once-luminous intrigue of his surroundings.

Yet, even as anger bubbled within him, DeCola found himself at a loss on how to convey his disillusionment to his primate performers. Their world, so detached from his own, seemed unaffected by the human expressions of discontent. The monkeys, engrossed in their gymnastic ballet, appeared oblivious to DeCola's changing moods, their focus undeterred by the audience's reception.

In a moment of unexpected revelation, DeCola found himself at a pivotal crossroads, standing at the outskirts of the bizarre city that had been the stage for his strange adventures. Fueled by a deep-seated desire to return to the realm of familiarity, he faced the direction he believed would lead him home, his heart heavy with uncertainty.

In a moment hovering on the edge of the unknown, De-Cola found himself whispering desires for closure on this bewildering journey. Gazing towards what he believed was the heart of this enigmatic world, he yearned for a glimpse of the city's core, a place he imagined would hold unparalleled beauty. These murmurs to himself, borne out of a deep-seated need to change the scene, were more potent than he realized.

As he focused on the path ahead, imbued with a mix of determination and a dash of resignation, something extraordinary happened. DeCola felt an unexpected surge, a gentle yet insistent force propelling him toward his desired destination. This sudden shift in momentum was startling, a stark contrast to the controlled movements he had grown accustomed to.

In this instant of unanticipated autonomy, DeCola experienced a profound shock. The realization washed over him like a wave, illuminating the truth that had eluded him: his will, an intrinsic force he barely recognized, held the power to surmount the external control he had been subjected to. This internal revelation was an incredible awakening in the fog of his ordeal, shedding light on the strength that resided within him, self-determination, a will that could defy the constraints of the misleading captives.

This unanticipated discovery, nestled within an un-guarded moment of self-reaction, was a turning point for De-Cola. It was a testament to the resilience of the human spirit, a reminder that even in the depths of manipulation and de-ceit, the essence of one's strong will could emerge victorious. As he moved, unencumbered, towards his goal, the shackles of his previous constraints seemed to dissolve, leaving him with a renewed sense of empowerment and the thrilling re-alization of his autonomous power.

DeCola's initial wonder and curiosity, the driving forces behind his long and tiresome journey, dissipated in the face of this harsh reality as he eventually arrived at the expected destination. The stark contrast between his expectations and the actuality of the destination filled him with a sense of be-trayal and an emotional questioning of the journey's purpose. This was not a place where a person with the slightest incli-nation towards civility and order could find solace or a sense of belonging. It was, in every conceivable way, the antithesis of what he had been led to believe he would find. Contrary to his expectations, the habitation was an unwelcoming and distasteful end - a bitter pill to swallow. It was a moment that underscored the unpredictable nature of his adventure, a touching reminder that the pursuit of the unknown could sometimes lead to places far removed from the realms of desirable comfort.

DeCola's journey, fraught with confusion and manipulation, culminated in a profound disillusionment as he arrived at what was supposed to be the climax of his extraordinary voyage. The anticipation of discovering a utopian city, a place of unparalleled beauty and harmony, crumbled away to reveal a starkly different reality. The destination that lay before him was a far cry from the idyllic visions he had conjured in his mind. Instead, he was met with a scene of chaos and squalor, an environment so jarringly disorderly and filthy that it struck a chord of deep dismay within him.

Upon arrival, DeCola was confronted with a scene that defied any notion of beauty or civility he had harbored, far from the utopian city he had envisioned. The environment that unfolded before him was an indication of chaos and neglect. It was as if the very essence of disorder had taken physical form, manifesting in a settlement that was not just uninviting but profoundly repulsive.

The habitation was a jarring integration of squalor and disarray, an affront to the senses that left DeCola fretting. The dirt that clung to every surface seemed almost crusty, a testament to the neglect that permeated the place. The bizarre nature of the settlement extended to its inhabitants. They were unappealing, a collection of beings peculiar to the monkeys he recently encountered in the jungle, which seemed to have been conjured from a nightmare. The sight of the settlers only served to amplify the sense of alienation and dismay that washed over DeCola.

It was not a world of wonders of enlightened beings; it was a domain of degradation, a place where the very concept of civility is non-existent. The stark contrast between DeCola's aspirations for this journey and the grim reality he encountered marked a profound moment of disillusionment. The destination he had reached, far from being a pinnacle of achievement or discovery, was opposed to everything he valued and desired. The disappointment that overshadowed DeCola was not just about the unlivable conditions or the unsettling nature of its dwellers. It was a profound disillusionment that the climax of the journey itself and the realization that the destination would be worthwhile was nothing but a facade. The hope and intrigue that had once propelled him forward had given way to a disappointing stark reality, leaving him to grapple with the bitter truth of his misguided adventurous gamble.

As DeCola arrived at the entrance of what was then revealed to him as "Regretopia: The City of Mischievous Mockery", the sight that greeted him was chilling to the bone. A massive, filthy banner loomed overhead, its letters crudely daubed in what appeared to be blood, proclaiming a sinister welcome to all who dared enter. The gatekeepers, clad in vile garb that seemed to merge with their equally unsettling manner, required no introduction from him. With a mere gesture, they conveyed their creepy anticipation of his arrival, their actions shrouded in a silent understanding that chilled DeCola to his core.

In an unexpected twist, DeCola's guide through this daunting city was to be a gargantuan parrot, its feathers disheveled and bearing the look of many untold stories. With an air of resignation, DeCola steeled himself to follow this unlikely escort, marveling at the bird's formidable presence as it launched into the air. The parrot's wingbeats filled the silence, and soon, it began to communicate in a manner that transcended the boundaries of human and avian speech.

To DeCola's bewilderment and slight annoyance, every squawk, chirp, and melodramatic sigh from the oversized parrot was translated directly into his brainwaves, a bizarre twist that had him questioning the very fabric of reality. The absurdity of receiving crystal-clear, bird-delivered commentary in his language left him oscillating between disbelief and begrudging respect for the digital chip's unexpected capabilities. As he trailed behind this feathered narrator, DeCola couldn't help but brace himself for what this comedic tour through the City of Regretopia might unveil, all while grappling with the weird experience of being guided by a parrot that seemed to have swallowed a GPS.

As the journey through Regretopia unfolded, led by the parrot with its mysterious device dictating directions like an old sea captain, DeCola was introduced to the city's seven unattractive landmarks. Each one, hilariously enough, seemed to be an exaggerated reaction to his inner turmoil, turning the tour into what felt like an elaborate amplification of his struggles. The precision with which these spots mirrored his trials was unmistakable, almost as if the parrot was a part comedian and part psychic, poking fun at his emotional expense with every turn of the journey.

DeCola's trip through Regretopia, with a drama-queen parrot as his guide, was like a wild ride through a theme park of ups and downs.

— First, they hit Peak Pessimism, where the mood changed faster than a light switch – one second, it's all sunny. The next, it's a total downpour.

— Next, they splashed into the Waters of Worry. Picture a pool where, instead of water, it was filled with shreds of doubts adjacent to the Shields of Self-Esteem, which are more like leaky floaties.

— Then, it was off to the Plains of Postponement, basically a giant couch where the Slothful Pandas hung out, putting off everything till "later." The Map of Motivation was used as a mat.

— The Ridges of Distress were up next, where making mountains out of molehills was the main sport, and the Anxiety Ants were the champs. The Giant Leaf of Perspective? Buried under a pile of worries.

— The Maze of Melancholy was the spot where a man was stuck in an insulated enclosure and his echo is the only friend, and within, the Shadow Selves jump out for a scare when you least expect it.

— Down in the Depths of Despair, concealed in the Hollows of Gloom, was a full-blown disaster movie soundtrack, ordinarily launched by a tiny hiccup, then amplified by sinister Loudspeakers.

— The last stop, the Island of Self-surrender, where giving up was the name of the game. Wearing the Armor of Achievement felt like dressing up in a suit of "I can't do this," and the Crown of Confidence was way too tight.

With each eccentric spot, the parrot announced, DeCola just had to keep going, turning his journey into an ominous orientation through the symbolic trials of Regretopia. It wasn't so much a profound quest as it was a rage-worthy stumble through a land of over-the-top troubles.

Through its shadowed corners, a crooked path laden with heavy stones of sorrow and regret, the parrot, with the hauntingly accurate narration, led DeCola through the heart of Regretopia, each named location, a reaction of the trials that lay in wait. This journey through the twisted terrains of Regretopia, with its landmarks of lament, offered not an enlightenment but a burdensome insight into the inner self.

As DeCola's tour of Regretopia took a turn from whimsical to wearisome, he couldn't shake off the feeling that he had become the target of an elaborate joke. Grumbling to himself, he reached his limit with the shenanigans. Fueled by his growing exasperation, a thought flashed in his mind to give the parrot guide, the ringmaster of this peculiar carnival, a knock-out punch.

Yet, he quickly reminded himself of the peculiar nature of his circumstances. Engaging in a confrontation with a guide that seemed more than meets the eye was probably not the wisest course of action. After all, there was the overwhelming sensation that his every move, even his thoughts, was under constant surveillance.

Just as DeCola entertained a fleeting wish for the parrot to experience a harmful tumble from the sky, the bird paused, turned to face him with apprehension, and delivered a stern caution: "If you dare turn your wish into a will or express it in words, you will surely die." It was as if the bird had telepathically intercepted his frustrated thought, warning him against harboring such wishes with an unfriendly stern and yet thought-provoking admonition.

This unexpected reprimand left DeCola in a state of confusion. He had often nursed the idea of suicide in the past if that would put an end to his sufferings. Nonetheless, he has come to understand that the whole scenario indicated that getting rid of the body does not solve the puzzle of suffering beyond his demise in the realms of the invisible – spirits, angels, or demons, whatever they are called or known by. Initially, DeCola had been led to believe that he had become so powerful with far-reaching eternal capabilities. Yet, here was this avian admonisher, that he is not immune to death after all. The contradictions were baffling. Whatever he settles for, he concludes that the malign forces that mean no good are not worthy of being listened to as they are obviously misleading. This truth is reinforced by the full understanding that he possesses the strong will to disobey them by choice.

Reacting to the caution of the bird of misfortune, DeCola circumstantially opted for prudence. He chose to remain silent, even though he was convinced that navigating the strangeness of Regretopia required a healthy dose of skepticism. It appeared that in this land of oddities, taking anything at face value was a venture into the absurd.

In the wake of his newfound autonomy, DeCola was besieged by doubts regarding the supposed extraordinary status conferred upon him through cerebral surgery. The realization that he possessed control over his movements led him to scrutinize the narrative of the embedded chip. He pondered the true origin of his debilitating headaches, questioning the absence of surgical evidence. This introspection led him to consider a more mundane yet sinister possibility: that his captors might have inflicted a blunt physical trauma, fabricating the tale of surgery of embedding a controlling device to manipulate his perception and necessitate submission as they take control.

With a mix of defiance and curiosity, he commanded his unseen mode of transportation to ascend higher into the sky, and it obeyed. Each subsequent command to alter course or altitude was met with compliance, reinforcing his belief in his control over the situation. This series of successful commands was a turning point for DeCola, a clear indication that the reins of power were, indeed, in his hands.

Armed with this revelation, DeCola's resolve hardened. He was determined to disregard any future commands from the once-dominant voice, a voice he no longer trusted. The path home was unclear, shrouded in uncertainty, but DeCola was ready to embrace the challenge, relying solely on his instincts and newfound autonomy. The thrill of piloting his invisible aircraft, free from external control, was a reference to his indomitable will.

Finally, DeCola's journey, fueled by constant determination, brought him back to the familiar streets and faces of his local community. This return, bathed in the soft light of renewed understanding, brought him to the doorstep of what once was his sanctuary. Yet, amidst the warmth of home fires and the gentle murmur of family life, DeCola remains adrift, a voyager returned yet not quite anchored. The familial bonds, once the melody to which his heart beats, now seem like a song half-remembered, leaving him in a puzzle on how to rekindle connections that once defined his essence.

His recent experience catalyzed a drastic shift in DeCola's worldview. The betrayal he felt, compounded by the realization of his manipulated perception, added to the caricature of his prevalent condition mirrored within Regretopia by a bizarre bird led him to adopt a cynical stance against other humans later. The world, in his eyes, became a stage for deceivers, a dwelling of the grossly insensitive, a place where trust was a commodity too precious to squander lightly. This skepticism extended to all, as DeCola vowed to take nothing at face value, guided by the belief that only his will was reliable, whether it was influenced by internal machinations or expressed by his genuine self. Nonetheless, he also realized he was not a perfect being and may still need help, anyway.

Since DeCola's ordeal began, he found himself entangled in a web of sleep and virtual experiences, uncertain whether these adventures unfolded in slumber or the waking world. His family, treading lightly, rarely disturbed his rest, aware of his aversion to being roused. DeCola harbored a strong belief in his right to undisturbed sleep, reducing his feeding and hydrating activities and causing him to lose more weight.

Navigating the blurred lines between his extraordinary journey and reality proved challenging for DeCola. He struggled to pinpoint when his fantastical experiences intersected with his interactions with family, if at all. Time lost its significance to him, and attempts to engage with his loved ones only heightened his irritability, deepening more isolation.

With some inward modulation, DeCola still lingered in a strange world, navigating through invisible currents that had once bound him and yet afloat by the conviction that he was the master of his destiny. This paradigm shift, from being a puppet of an unseen force to the captain of his ship, marked a significant chapter in DeCola's story, one where the lines between reality and perception, control and freedom, were irrevocably unclear. What a change!

Chapter 4: The Turning Point

Sustained by this newfound, albeit fragile, resolve, De-Cola embarked on the daunting odyssey of seeking help. The initial steps were hesitant, laden with the heavy chains of stigma and the echoes of society's whispers that to seek help was to reveal weakness. Each attempt to navigate the intricate maze of the mental health care system felt akin to traversing an ever-shifting landscape, where clarity was obscured by bureaucratic fog and the silhouettes of unending paperwork.

In the complexity of DeCola's life, woven with threads of routine and resilience, a single thread began to sparkle with the promise of change. This thread, seemingly inconspicuous at first, was to become the beacon that guided De-Cola through the darkest corridors of his mind toward a light he had almost ceased to believe in. The phenomenon unfolds as the narrative arc bends towards hope, marking the dawn of "The Turning Point."

The self-realization wasn't immediate but rather a slow dawning, like the first light of dawn creeping across a darkened landscape. It was born from countless moments of frustration, where his coping mechanisms faltered, leaving him feeling more isolated and helpless. The acknowledgment of his limitations, though humbling, was also a pivotal turning point.

DeCola's initial reluctance to seek help was rooted in a mixture of fears, misconceptions, and distrust. Aside, the fear of stigma, of being labeled or misunderstood, had long cast a shadow over the prospect of reaching out. Yet, the weight of his struggle began to nudge him toward the realization that the path to healing often requires a variety of support.

"The Turning Point" marks the chapter where the narrative shifts from a descent into despair to an ascent toward hope and healing. It is here that DeCola, guided by the contingent light of a rekindled friendship and the shared stories of struggle and strength, takes the first courageous step toward a future where the promise of change becomes a tangible possibility. This chapter is a testament to the power of connection, the strength found in vulnerability, and the profound impact that a single moment of genuine human interaction can have on the curve of our lives.

DeCola began to see the value in non-professional support, in the strength that can be drawn from the shared experiences of peers, the comfort of family, and the understanding of friends. He recognized that while professional guidance was crucial, the journey of healing was multifaceted, enriched by the empathy, perspectives, and companionship of a wider support network.

This shift in perspective enhanced DeCola's inclination for professional support from which others like him have benefited, giving the expertise of those trained to navigate the web of mental health more room. Nevertheless, the thought of opening up to a stranger, of laying bare his vulnerabilities, still lingered. However, the promise of understanding, of strategies tailored to his unique experience, began to chip away at the walls he had built around himself.

The decision to embrace both professional and non-professional support marked a new chapter in DeCola's journey, one characterized by collaboration rather than isolation. It was a step towards building a bridge between his inner world and the external support systems available to him, a bridge that promised to lead him toward a more hopeful horizon.

This vital moment was not about surrender but about empowerment, a conscious choice to harness every available resource in his quest for well-being. As DeCola tentatively reached out, taking those first steps towards seeking help, he set in motion a transformative process, one that would not only redefine his path to recovery but also reshape his understanding of strength, vulnerability, and the power of connection.

This openness armed DeCola with an eagerness to involve the relevant intervention team which he had earlier dismissed. He was encouraged about the role of the intervention encompassing the methods used to support individuals experiencing events that produce emotional, mental, physical, and behavioral distress or problems, focusing on a pragmatic and exhaustive approach to crisis intervention involving a concerted team of professionals.

DeCola's Quest for the Right Strategy

DeCola's journey through professional intervention for his complex mental health issues was anything but ordinary, marked by a series of comically unexpected interruptions that tested the adaptability of his care team. He was encouraged to attend initial preliminary workshops and training of his choice to give the professionals some idea about how best to support him. Despite the gravity of his situation, DeCola regained his innate tendency for entertainment as he resolved to engage the professionals and turned many a therapeutic session into an impromptu comedy show.

During one particularly solemn counseling session aimed at unpacking his feelings, DeCola suddenly burst into an operatic rendition of his woes, turning the room into a makeshift stage. His therapists caught off guard but ever resourceful, decided to roll with it, turning the session into a musical exploration of emotions, much to everyone's amusement.

For instance, in group therapy, DeCola once decided that the arrangement of chairs was too conventional, prompting him to rearrange the furniture into what he deemed a more "energetically favorable" spiral formation. This unexpected interior redesign led to an impromptu discussion on personal space and boundaries, providing valuable insights most unconventionally.

During a mindfulness exercise meant to foster a sense of calm, DeCola misinterpreted the instructions and ended up leading the group in what can only be described as a stand-up comedy routine about the absurdities of daily life. The laughter that ensued broke down barriers among the participants, fostering a sense of togetherness and mutual understanding.

Art therapy sessions with DeCola were never dull. Tasked with expressing his feelings through paint, he took it upon himself to critique everyone's artwork in the style of a flamboyant self-appointed art judge, complete with dramatic pauses and exaggerated gestures such as waving both hands in the air. This unexpected art critique session turned into a lesson on perspective-taking and constructive feedback, much to the delight of all involved.

The professionals working with DeCola, recognizing the therapeutic value hidden within his odd disruptions, skillfully incorporated his unique expressions into the intervention process. They used humor as a bridge to deeper understanding, demonstrating the importance of flexibility and creativity in mental health care. Through these lively and often hilarious interactions, DeCola's journey became a testament to the healing power of laughter and the human capacity to find light even in the darkest of times.

To ensure a successful intervention tailored to DeCola's unique needs, the main team of professionals decided to hold an initial meeting with him after confirming that all professionals had fully read and understood his recorded story. This meeting was designed to be inclusive, empathetic, and focused on DeCola's specific situation, ensuring his active participation in the planning process. DeCola was fully informed, and his consent was sought for the crucial meeting.

As DeCola prepared for his initial encounter with the team of professionals, the air was thick with anticipation. The team, a diverse group comprising a counselor, a medical doctor, a Dietitian, a social worker, and the care coordinator, huddled together beforehand to strategize. Their goal was clear: to speak DeCola's language, both literally and metaphorically, and to foster an atmosphere where he felt at ease.

In their briefing, they reviewed DeCola's file, careful not to jump to conclusions. They knew the importance of seeing DeCola, the person, beyond DeCola, the case. As they discussed their approach, they emphasized patience, clarity, and empathy, preparing to meet DeCola wherever he was on his journey.

DeCola was eager to make a grand entrance, complete with unscheduled intermissions and an array of comic tales. The team of professionals displayed the patience of saints, waiting with the serene composure of those well-versed in the unpredictable rhythms of their client's lives. Their early arrival and preparedness set a professional tone of dedication and understanding that even DeCola's flamboyant disruptions couldn't unsettle.

As DeCola finally made his appearance, fashionably late and with the air of a seasoned performer, the team greeted him with warm smiles and an air of genuine interest that seemed to cushion the room. The atmosphere was devoid of clinical coldness; instead, it was infused with a sense of ingenuity and more, as if welcoming an old friend rather than a case number.

The moment DeCola stepped into the room, the dynamics shifted. With unexpectedly comedic timing, DeCola broke the ice not with a handshake but with a bewildering anecdote about his morning encounter with a "telepathic squirrel which instructed him on how to read people's minds." He adds, "…be careful about your personal opinions of me!". The professionals caught off guard, couldn't help but chuckle, nodding their heads in agreement, their well-laid plans momentarily derailed by DeCola's unpredictable humor.

Nonetheless, DeCola's unexpected outburst of laughter cut through the warm welcome like a sharp knife; expressing his sudden anger pointed directly at a decorative picture hanging behind the team. Through his giggles, he managed to articulate his suspicion, "I'm not naive, am I? Or is this some kind of setup?" What caught DeCola's eye was a peculiar painting that depicted a funny scene – a group of cartoon animals engaged in what appeared to be a therapy session, with a wise-looking owl in the center, donning spectacles and holding a clipboard. To DeCola, this seemed like a thinly veiled jab, a caricature of his recent experience, which set off alarm bells in his head.

The meeting coordinator, sensing DeCola's discomfort and understanding the potential for misinterpretation, quickly stepped in to clarify with a calming smile. "Ah, that painting," the coordinator began with a light-hearted chuckle, "It's actually an old piece the clinic staff found at a local art fair. It's meant to add a touch of humor and lightness to the room. We understand how sessions can sometimes feel daunting, and a little fun can go a long way."

The coordinator continued, "We assure you, DeCola, there's no hidden agenda here. Our sole focus is your well-being and comfort. We chose this artwork to remind everyone not to take things too seriously all the time and to create an environment where laughter can be part of the healing process."

Tickled by the coordinator's smooth handling of the mix-up, DeCola seized the moment for some dramatic air. With an exquisite gesture fitting for the theatre and a voice dripping with simulated significance, he stepped into the spotlight. "In that case, Ladies and gentlemen," he announced, a spark of playful cunning in his gaze, "I present to you DeCola, the unexpected champion, battling relentless cosmic invaders and yet, here I stand, unvanquished!" His peculiar style of self-introduction was a tactic to convey to the team that he won't allow anyone to take him for a ride, an eye-opener into his personality.

The professionals, adept at navigating the diverse personalities that graced their practice, didn't miss a beat. They welcomed DeCola's self-introduction with a mix of applause and nods, their comportment blending professional respect with a touch of amusement at his unique approach. This seamless adjustment to DeCola's style set the stage for a meeting where hierarchy and formality took a backseat to empathy and connection, ensuring DeCola felt welcome as well as celebrated for his individuality.

Throughout the session, DeCola's witty interjections kept the team on their toes. From playful misinterpretations of medical terms to light-hearted impersonations of the "Mood Monitor Monkeys" he claimed were his advisors, DeCola infused the meeting with a unique blend of silliness and chaos.

The professionals, recognizing the therapeutic value of humor, skillfully wove DeCola's jests into the conversation, using them as springboards to delve deeper into his experiences. They navigated his comedic outbursts with grace, redirecting the energy toward constructive dialogue while ensuring DeCola felt heard and valued.

In this unexpected dance of dialogue, DeCola's humor became a bridge, connecting him with the team in a way that conventional methods might not have achieved. The meeting, though dotted with laughter, laid the groundwork for a relationship built on understanding, respect, and a shared appreciation for the lighter side of life, even in the face of adversity.

After the self-introduction of each of the participating professionals, the meeting coordinator, with a flourish of officialdom, announced that the entire intervention process would be crafted around DeCola's specific needs, explaining the meeting's goal in simple terms: "We're here to talk about how we can best support you through this tough time. We want to plan together. A plan that makes sense to you", dubbing it "DeCola's Model," DeCola couldn't help but puff up with pride. He sat up straighter, a grin spreading across his face as visions of his name in psychology textbooks danced in his head. "Finally," he thought, "I'm not just a participant; I'm the main event!" His reaction pleased the professionals as he approved their proposal.

When the team further outlined the collaborative approach to setting recovery goals, emphasizing the importance of DeCola's active involvement, he couldn't help but interject with a mix of disbelief and humor. "You're kidding me, right?" he said, chuckling. "So, you're telling me I get to be the captain of this ship? Next, you'll be saying I get to pick the pirate crew and the treasure map!"

The professionals, getting accustomed to DeCola's unique way of processing information, smiled at his analogy. They played along, affirming his pivotal role in the journey ahead. "Absolutely, Captain DeCola," the coordinator responded as the spokesperson: "Consider us your loyal crew, ready to navigate the high seas of recovery. Just don't make us walk the plank if we hit rough waters!"

DeCola, amused by the team's willingness to engage with his perspective, leaned into the narrative. "Alright, crew," he declared with a mock-serious tone, "let's chart a course for my strange adventure. I hope you are the actual solution to my long-standing struggles." he reacted.

This light-hearted exchange not only diffused the tension but also reinforced the message that DeCola's input was not just valued but essential. It underscored the team's commitment to a partnership where DeCola's voice led the way, with the professionals there to support and guide rather than dictate the course of his journey.

When the issue of mutual feedback and adjustments was raised at the earliest stage of recovery planning, DeCola injected a bit of humor into the serious conversation. He quipped, "So, feedback, huh? I always thought that was just what happens when sound echoes. But now you're telling me I get to echo back at you?" This light-hearted comment highlighted DeCola's understanding of the term 'feedback' in a literal sense before diving into its application in their context.

Continuing with his jest, DeCola playfully challenged the idea of adjustments, asking, "And adjustments... if I'm really in the driver's seat here, does that mean you'll be adjusting to me?" In a playful twist, he said, "Don't go tipping the script on me now!" ". He cleverly affirmed his privileged position, implying that if he were to lead the recovery process truly, it would be the professionals who might need to adapt to his feedback and preferences rather than the other way round.

Through this humorous exchange, DeCola acknowledged the team's effort to involve him actively in his care plan while also expressing his newfound sense of empowerment in a light-hearted manner. It underscored the shift from a traditional patient role to an active participant in the healthcare process, where his opinions and preferences would lead to mutual adjustments between him and the healthcare team to tailor the recovery plan to his needs.

The meeting unfolded with the precision of a well-rehearsed play, each professional taking their cue to contribute to what would become the content of his mental health intervention. The counselor kicked things off with a deep dive into DeCola's emotional landscape, navigating the peaks and valleys with the finesse of a seasoned mountaineer. DeCola, reveling in the spotlight, offered dramatic reenactments of his encounters with the Mood Monitor Monkeys, complete with interpretive dance.

During the discussion, as the team emphasized the virtues of active listening and empathy, DeCola raised his hand like a curious student in the middle of a particularly puzzling lecture. "Hold up," he interjected with a puzzled look, "What's this 'active listening' thing? Is that like listening with your whole body? Should I be wiggling my ears or something?"

The room paused, a smile tugging at the corners of the professionals' lips as they processed DeCola's unique take on the concept. Not missing a beat, DeCola continued, "And empathy – is that like feeling sorry for someone but in a fancy way?"

The coordinator, seizing the opportunity to bridge De-Cola's colorful interpretations with the essence of the concepts, responded with a twinkle in his eye. "Well, DeCola, active listening might not require ear gymnastics, but it's all about tuning in with your heart and mind, really hearing what someone's saying beyond the words. And as for empathy, it's more like putting yourself in someone else's shoes, even if they're clown shoes, and dancing a mile in them."

DeCola, nodding sagely, back, "Ah, so it's like listening with my soul and feeling with their feet. Got it!" The room erupted in gentle laughter, appreciating DeCola's jovial and yet insightful interpretation. The coordinator cleverly acknowledged DeCola's perspective, weaving it into the fabric of their approach and ensuring that the concepts of active listening and empathy were not just explained but lived out in their interaction.

As the medical doctor rose to discuss DeCola's health, DeCola couldn't resist turning the moment into a scene straight out of a comedy sketch. "Hey, aren't you my GP?" he blurted out, his voice dripping with mock surprise as all eyes snapped at him. "Quite hysterical - I dreamt I saw you at the zoo, being chased by this furious ostrich! Man, you should've seen yourself sprinting; I had no idea you were such an athlete. And you, a doctor, didn't even dare to calm down a single bird with a tranquilizer?"

The room fell into hushed anticipation, everyone bracing for the GP's response, wondering if the professional atmosphere was about to take a nosedive. But the GP, gathered himself together with a twinkle of amusement in his eye, smoothly retorted, "I appreciate your humorous dream and vivid imagination, DeCola. In your dream, I might be dodging ostriches, but be rest assured, in reality, I'm here as your dedicated human GP, not a vet."

This amusing comeback not only diffused the tension but also drew a collective chuckle from the room. DeCola, delighted by the doctor's sportive engagement, nodded approvingly, his respect for the GP's professional and mature handling of the situation visibly growing. The exchange, while jokey, underscored the mutual understanding and rapport building between DeCola and his care team, setting a positive tone for the rest of the discussion.

Recognizing the importance of maintaining focus amidst DeCola's humorous interjections, the GP skillfully steered the conversation back to the matter at hand. With a blend of professionalism and tact, he succinctly delivered his presentation, ensuring that every crucial detail regarding DeCola's physical well-being and clinical history was communicated clearly. The GP's prudent approach ensured that the essential information was not lost in the laughter and provided DeCola and the team with the vital knowledge needed to proceed effectively. His ability to balance humor with the seriousness of medical discussion exemplified his commitment to DeCola's care without compromising the integrity of the consultation.

The social worker explored DeCola's environment and support system, mapping out a social network that, according to DeCola, included an advisory council of squirrels and pigeons. The team nodded along, their professional demeanor cracking slightly at DeCola's descriptions of pigeon-led group therapy sessions.

At the dietician's turn, she stepped in with a blend of expertise and warmth. She was ready to address DeCola's journey toward wellness. "Good day, DeCola," she began, her tone both friendly and informative, "I'm here to be your guide through the world of nutrition, crafting a map for your meals that not only tantalizes your physical taste buds but also fortifies your mental fortress". At that point, the dietician promptly noticed DeCola's raised eyebrows as soon as she described herself as a guide and tantalizing taste buds. Having meticulously read DeCola's clinical file and understood DeCola's narrated experience, and realizing the connection of her expression with the poetic verse that earlier misled DeCola at the peak of his mental health crisis, she quickly allays his fears by letting DeCola know that the choice of what he eats would be his exclusive right as no one would force anything on him or conceal any unwanted offer. She added, "Together, we'll explore foods that fuel not just the body but also items that nourish the mind, ensuring each bite brings you a step closer to recovery. Let's embark on this delicious adventure towards a healthier and happier you." Thus consolidating a clear contrast.

The care coordinator, responsible for orchestrating the comprehensive strategy, presented a detailed guide to achieving overall health, named "The DeCola Wellness Plan." DeCola's excited contributions marked each phase of the plan, proposing side trips to explore these mythical places.

As the clock ticked closer to lunchtime, the meeting coordinator, beaming with pride at the morning's progress, declared, "And now, dear colleagues, we've arrived at our scheduled time for recession." Before the last syllable could echo in the room, DeCola, ever the vigilant listener, jumped in with a bewildered frown. "Hold on, recession? In here, too? Are we going to start budget cuts on coffee and sandwiches now? Is no place safe from this economic doom and gloom? When do we begin to bloom?" he exclaimed, throwing his hands up in mock despair. "Next thing you know, they'll be taxing our bathroom breaks!"

The room caught between confusion and amusement, turned to the coordinator for clarification. With a gentle smile and a chuckle, the coordinator quickly cleared the air. "My apologies again for the mix-up, DeCola. I meant 'recess' as in a break for lunch, not 'recession' as in the economic term. No budget cuts here, I promise, and your coffee is safe!" The clarification brought a collective sigh of relief and a round of laughter as DeCola, now amused at his misunderstanding, led the charge to the lunch table, jokingly checking for any hidden austerity measures.

DeCola's Quest for Collaboration

As the team of professionals settled back in their seats after lunch, DeCola seized the moment before the coordinator could even get a word in. With an air for the dramatic, he leaped to his feet, striking a pose reminiscent of a seasoned theatre actor about to deliver a monologue. The room erupted in laughter as he dramatically announced, "Ladies and gentlemen, prepare yourselves for the grand act two!" His unexpected antics, which elicited a resounding applause, broke the ice again, setting a light-hearted tone for the afternoon session.

While the room echoed with laughter, DeCola playfully mentioned his older brother, who had quietly been waiting outside. "Just so you know, my big brother's out there, diving into his favorite budget snacks. I barred him from joining us—he's just too easy-going, always taking my word as law," he joked. While his comment seemed light-hearted, it revealed a close-knit sibling relationship. The team, careful not to endorse any seemingly negative remarks, managed to restrain their laughter, maintaining a respectful atmosphere.

However, the mood shifted slightly when one of the professionals decided to address DeCola's disregard for his brother gently. Her approach was thoughtful, aiming to offer a different perspective without offending. "You know, during our break, I stepped outside and had the chance to meet someone very interesting," she began, her voice warm, inviting everyone into the story she was about to tell. "He introduced himself as your brother, and honestly, I found his company quite delightful. He exuded this genuine warmth and seemed really invested in how things were going in here for you."

She continued, her narrative skillfully highlighting the brother's deep care and concern for DeCola, "He spoke so highly of you and seemed to be here purely out of a desire to support you. It's not often you come across such selflessness. It really made me appreciate the bond you two must share." Her words painted a picture of DeCola's brother not as the pushover DeCola had humorously branded him but as an epitome of unwavering support and love, subtly reshaping the narrative in a way that honored the depth of their familial ties.

Through this diplomatic approach, the professional not only acknowledges the brother's caring nature but also indirectly invites DeCola to reconsider his perspective on his deeply compassionate brother. By highlighting the brother's supportive presence as a sign of strength and love rather than weakness, she cleverly reacted to DeCola's delusion, provoking a more empathetic and appreciative understanding within DeCola without direct contradiction or offense.

After the meeting wrapped up, the team presented DeCola with a summary of the plan agreed upon, stripped of all the usual corporate gibberish. It was clear, concise, and re-freshingly free of terms that would make you want to look up a clinical dictionary. DeCola, with his unique blend of humor and sharp wit, couldn't help but quip, "So, what you're telling me is, we're actually going to understand what we're doing for once?" This light-hearted jest set a positive tone and underscored his appreciation for the straightforward ap-proach.

To keep the lines of communication as open as the skies using one of DeCola's favorite cartoons, the team handed him a list of direct contacts. Each name came with a little caricature, adding a personal touch that spoke to DeCola's comical side. "Ah, so if I need to summon the cavalry, I just use these magical incantations, huh?" he joked, pretending to wave a wand over the contact list. His playful acknowl-edgment of the open-door policy underscored the im-portance of easy access to the team for any clarifications or concerns.

The cherry on top was the scheduling of a follow-up meeting. It wasn't just any penciled-in appointment but a commitment to ensuring the plan didn't just sit collecting dust on a shelf. DeCola, ever the master of amusing compar-isons, likened it to a TV series, saying, "So, we're all set for the next episode, then? I'll bring the popcorn!" His light-hearted take on the follow-up schedule was a pointer to the power of collaboration and the continuous effort to nurture the budding partnership.

With a seamless transition, the team promptly underscores their commitment to DeCola's immediate needs. They meticulously identify with him where he is and are well prepared to ride alongside in a tender embrace of integrated care, signaling that he wasn't just another case but a valued individual whose peace of mind was their paramount concern. They were confidently accompanying him to a sanctuary within their space, a haven designed for comfort and candid conversation, ensuring he felt shielded even in the middle of chaos. In this nurturing cocoon, DeCola found himself undergoing a comprehensive wellness check, spanning head to toe, inside and out. This holistic approach, touching on the physical and the psychological, captures a clear picture of his overall health needs. DeCola, touched by the meticulous and heartfelt strategy, couldn't help but nod in agreement, a smile breaking through. The team's proposal, woven with care and expertise, felt like a tailored suit, fitting him perfectly and marking the beginning of a journey he was eager to embark on. Beyond abstract hope, he was fully empowered for the transformative healthcare adventure.

Something seems to work out the magic for DeCola. The team purposefully reached out to him, combining urgency with a warm, compassionate touch that resonated deeply with him. This swift action showed DeCola he was a top priority and his wellbeing mattered greatly. They also made sure the setting was safe and comfortable, creating an atmosphere that encouraged open dialogue and made DeCola feel so secure. Furthermore, the team prioritizes DeCola's needs, be it physical, medical, or psychological, along with a series of relevant tests to ensure his overall health is addressed at the right time. DeCola was visibly moved by the team's thorough and empathetic approach, wholeheartedly approving their proposed actions with a smile grateful for the genuine concern and support they extended towards him.

Quick to voice his concern, DeCola piped up, "Don't skip the brain check, yeah? That's where all the trouble's at for me." His GP responded with a smile, "You're right on target, DeCola!" He laid out the plan, mentioning that a sit-down with both a psychologist and a psychiatrist was already on the books for a deep dive into what was happening in DeCola's head, which may lead to further scans, weighing all clinical implications. In addition, the doctor explained how the team would involve DeCola's family to ensure the desired support is received to enhance his recovery. The GP further prepared DeCola for more help that may be needed along the way with the flexibility to adjust the plans when necessary to suit DeCola, making sure to keep things straightforward as they jointly moved forward.

With a burst of genuine enthusiasm, DeCola couldn't help but exclaim, "Wow, I really dig how you all are dotting the i's and crossing the t's! You're thorough, men, and I like that!" spirited approval filled the room, reacting his growing confidence in the team's comprehensive approach.

Moving seamlessly into a deeper understanding of DeCola's situation, the team harnessed the power of empathy and careful listening. They tuned into his narrative with unwavering attention, creating a space where DeCola felt truly heard. Every word he shared was met with nods of understanding as the team skillfully mirrored his thoughts back to him, stripping away any jargon that could become the essence of their communication. In this exchange, DeCola's strengths and moments of resilience weren't just acknowledged; they were celebrated, shining a light on his innate ability to navigate through storms. This approach not only fortified the bond between DeCola and the team but also kindled a spark of confidence within him, a sense that, perhaps, he was indeed equipped to weather the storm. DeCola, feeling both understood and valued, couldn't help but beam with approval, silently commending the team's insightful and respectful handling of his story.

Recapturing comprehensive assessment, the team cast a wide net at the full spectrum of DeCola's condition, touching on the physical, social, emotional, and mental facets of his well-being. They navigated the sensitive terrain with a gentle touch, making sure DeCola felt at ease to peel back the layers of his life's story. The conversation took an uplifting turn as the team wove in empowering questions, sparking in DeCola's thoughts of what lies ahead, his values, and the kind of support he dreamed of. This shift towards the positive not only painted a bright horizon but also placed DeCola in the driver's seat of his journey to wellness.

The team shifted their focus to fostering a sense of empowerment within DeCola, urging him to play a leading role in shaping the intervention plan. This approach struck a chord with DeCola, feeding his determination and solidifying his investment in the recovery process. As the session ended, the team wrapped up with an uplifting message carefully crafted to resonate with DeCola's unique passions and dreams. Their steadfast confidence in his ability to overcome the challenges ahead, coupled with their commitment to stand by him, ignited a spark of inspiration in DeCola. He left the meeting not just content but energized, ready to tackle the path to wellness with a newfound zeal.

As the initial phase of intervention ended, "DeCola's Model" evolved from a standard intervention plan into a vibrant tapestry of creativity, humor, and genuine care. The team, initially bewildered by DeCola's antics, found themselves invigorated by the challenge of weaving his unique perspective into their approach. The team truly honored their commitment to support and collaboration. In wrapping up the section, they turned to DeCola, inquiring if he had any questions or needed further explanations about what had been discussed.

This gesture underscored their dedication to transparency and ensuring DeCola's understanding and comfort with the process. Moreover, they reiterated their promise of ongoing support and the willingness to adapt the plan as needed, emphasizing the dynamic and responsive nature of the support they were offering. This approach not only reinforced the collaborative spirit they pledged to uphold but also cemented a foundation of trust and mutual respect as they moved forward with the intervention.

DeCola's initial planning meeting was like a comedy sketch set in an otherworldly fantasy. Picture this: he described the team as if they were a quirky band of wizards and mystics straight out of a fairy tale, each armed with a spell book of recovery strategies. DeCola, the accidental hero of this tale, found himself in what felt like a magical summit, expecting a dragon to crash the meeting with every wellness tip. As he joked about how he was navigating the 'enchanted' gathering as he described it, he asked the team regarding how he had performed. The team rated him well, acknowledging how he impressed them with his helpful participation giving him a resounding applause.

In his hilariously skewed version of events, routine suggestions transformed into epic quests, and the exchange of feedback turned into whimsical banter with creatures of lore. Despite the layers of humor and a pinch of delightful delusion with hallucinatory undertones, he managed to capture the spirit of the team's efforts in his own unusual, laughter-filled way, proving that humor can be the most enchanting bridge between understanding and imagination.

DeCola, for his part, left the meeting feeling like a celebrity, convinced that "DeCola's Model" would revolutionize the field. The professionals, amused and inspired by DeCola's unorthodox contributions, recognized the value of infusing their work with a dose of humor, acknowledging that the path to healing is not just through the mind but through the heart and laughter, too.

As the meeting ended, a palpable sense of fulfillment enveloped the room. The team and DeCola exchanged looks of mutual respect and accomplishment, their faces alight with the shared success of a well-conducted session. With a sense of ceremony, they rose from their seats, and the air buzzed with the promise of the journey ahead.

As the meeting ended, a palpable sense of accomplishment enveloped the room, like the final chords of a symphony resonating with both the performers and the audience. The team and DeCola exchanged glances, each pair of eyes sparkling with the shared knowledge of a job well begun. With smiles as bright as the morning sun, they rose from their seats, the air humming with positive energy. With a surge of renewed optimism, DeCola reached out and extended his hand with a flourish, engaging in hearty handshakes that spoke volumes more than words ever could, evidence of more confidence and trust he had gained. His spirit was lit and lifted. Each clasp was firm and warm, sealing the unspoken pact of mutual dedication toward the journey ahead. The atmosphere had transformed into a cocoon of camaraderie, the handshakes serving as a clear demonstration of a meeting that had sown the seeds of hope and anticipation for the transformative days to come.

Chapter 5: Embracing Vulnerability

In this chapter, DeCola stands at the precipice of a profound revelation: the power inherent in vulnerability, the sheer bravery it takes to expose one's true self, scars and all. As DeCola begins to peel back the layers of self-protection, they encounter the freeing sensation of authenticity, a state of being where the fear of judgment gives way to the possibility of genuine connection.

DeCola's decision to share their story marks a pivotal moment in their journey. It's an act that transcends the personal, challenging the pervasive stigma surrounding mental health. By speaking their truth, DeCola lights a beacon for others lost in the shadows of their struggles, signaling that it's not only okay not to be okay, but it's also okay to talk about it. This act of sharing becomes a key that unlocks doors to conversations that many fear to open, fostering a community where silence is replaced by dialogue and isolation by solidarity.

The chapter delves deep into the transformative impact of vulnerability on relationships. As DeCola navigates this new terrain of openness, they discover the profound depth of connection that vulnerability can foster. Friendships and familial bonds, once surface-level in their interactions, deepen into reservoirs of mutual support and understanding. DeCola finds that in showing their authentic self, others are encouraged to do the same, creating a virtuous cycle of sharing and empathy that enriches every interaction.

Moreover, embracing vulnerability propels DeCola's healing journey forward. It's in the moments of sharing their fears, hopes, and dreams that DeCola realizes the weight of the burdens they've been carrying alone. The act of verbalizing their experiences not only validates their feelings but also offers a new perspective on their struggles, seen through the lens of communal wisdom and support.

"Embracing Vulnerability" is a testament to the paradoxical strength found in openness and the power of vulnerability to transform not only the individual but also the communities they are a part of. This chapter celebrates the breaking down of walls, the shedding of facades, and the beauty of becoming truly seen. In DeCola's journey, we are reminded that it is through the courage to be vulnerable that we find our truest connections and the deepest wellspring of our strength.

DeCola's journey of embracing vulnerability and fostering resilience significantly contributes immensely to his mental health recovery, offering profound insights into the role of openness, perseverance, and authenticity in healing. Here is a systematic enumeration of how embracing vulnerability and resilience aids in DeCola's recovery:

DeCola Acknowledges His Struggles

DeCola's mental health recovery journey is fundamentally rooted in his ability to acknowledge his struggles himself, marking a pivotal moment of self-awareness and acceptance. This initial step of recognizing the reality of his mental health challenges is both profound and transformative, setting the stage for all subsequent steps in his healing process.

The act of acknowledgment serves as a gateway to vulnerability, enabling DeCola to confront the aspects of his life and psyche that he may have previously ignored or suppressed. This internal admission is not an easy task; it requires courage to face the discomfort and uncertainty that often accompany such realizations. However, it is this courage that catalyzes DeCola's journey toward recovery, breaking the chains of denial and isolation that can exacerbate mental health issues.

By acknowledging his struggles, DeCola shifts from a state of passive suffering to one of active engagement with his mental health. This shift is crucial, as it empowers him to take ownership of his journey, moving from a place of helplessness to one of agency. It opens the door to self-compassion, allowing DeCola to extend kindness and understanding to himself in the face of his challenges rather than succumbing to self-criticism or shame.

Furthermore, this acknowledgment is the first step in dismantling the stigma—both internal and societal—that often surrounds mental health issues. By admitting to himself that he is struggling, DeCola begins to erode the barriers of stigma, making it possible to reach out for help without the burden of judgment. This step is vital for seeking and receiving support, whether from friends, family, mental health professionals, or support groups.

The acknowledgment of his struggles also enhances DeCola's self-awareness, providing him with valuable insights into his needs, triggers, and coping mechanisms. This heightened awareness is instrumental in navigating the complexities of mental health recovery, enabling DeCola to identify what forms of support and intervention will be most beneficial for his unique situation.

In essence, DeCola's acknowledgment of his mental health struggles lays the groundwork for his recovery journey. It is a declaration of his readiness to embrace vulnerability, seek support, and embark on the path to healing. This foundational step not only propels DeCola forward in his journey but also serves as a powerful testament to the importance of self-acceptance and openness in the broader context of mental health recovery.

DeCola Challenges Stigma

DeCola's decision to embrace vulnerability and openly discuss his mental health experiences marks a pivotal moment in his recovery journey, serving as a powerful act of defiance against the stigma that often shrouds mental health. This deliberate choice to share his story not only propels his healing but also plays a significant role in fostering a societal shift toward greater acceptance and understanding of mental health issues.

By choosing to speak openly about his struggles and victories, DeCola confronts the pervasive stigma head-on, challenging the misconceptions and prejudices that can isolate individuals and discourage them from seeking help. His candidness helps dismantle the barriers of silence and shame that often surround mental health, encouraging a more open and empathetic dialogue within his community and beyond.

DeCola's vulnerability in sharing his journey serves as a beacon of solidarity, reaching out to others who may be suffering in silence. It sends a clear message that experiencing mental health challenges is not a sign of weakness but a part of the human condition that many navigate. This act of sharing creates a space for others to recognize their own experiences within his story, diminishing their sense of isolation and fostering a sense of shared humanity.

Moreover, DeCola's openness contributes to normalizing conversations about mental health, making it an integral part of everyday discussions, just like physical health. By incorporating his mental health experiences into his interactions, he helps others see mental well-being as an essential component of overall health, deserving of the same attention and care.

Furthermore, DeCola's challenge to mental health stigma extends beyond his immediate circle, influencing broader societal attitudes. Through public speaking engagements, social media, writing, or simply conversing with peers, his story becomes a tool for education, raising awareness about the complexities of mental health and the importance of support and compassion.

In essence, DeCola's active challenge to mental health stigma through embracing vulnerability and openness is a transformative aspect of his recovery. It not only aids in his healing journey but also contributes to building a more inclusive, empathetic, and understanding society. DeCola's story becomes a catalyst for change, inspiring others to break the silence around mental health and advocating for a world where mental well-being is embraced as a vital aspect of human life.

DeCola Joins Support Groups

DeCola's decision to join support groups marks a significant stride in his mental health recovery, harnessing the power of communal healing and shared experiences. This step, underscored by his willingness to embrace vulnerability, becomes a conduit for profound personal growth and connection.

Within the supportive confines of these groups, DeCola finds a unique space where stories and struggles, much like his own, are openly shared. This act of collective vulnerability creates a powerful bond among group members, forging a sense of solidarity and understanding that is often hard to find elsewhere. For DeCola, hearing the experiences of others not only validates his journey but also provides a broader perspective on the diverse ways individuals navigate mental health challenges.

As DeCola shares his narrative within the group, he contributes to this tapestry of shared experiences, adding his voice to the chorus of resilience and perseverance. This exchange is cathartic for DeCola, offering him a sense of relief and liberation as he unburdens his story in a space free from judgment. The act of vocalizing his journey, in turn, becomes a powerful tool for self-reflection and healing, helping him to process his experiences and gain insights into his path to recovery.

The support group also serves as a rich source of coping strategies and practical advice gleaned from the collective wisdom of its members. DeCola benefits from the diverse array of approaches and perspectives shared within the group, equipping him with new tools and techniques to manage his mental health. This exchange of knowledge is invaluable, providing DeCola with alternative solutions and viewpoints that he may not have considered on his own.

Moreover, the support group fosters a sense of belonging for DeCola, alleviating feelings of isolation that often accompany mental health struggles. Being part of a community that understands and shares similar experiences reassures him that he is not alone in his journey. This sense of belonging is integral to DeCola's recovery, as it bolsters his confidence and motivation to continue navigating the complexities of mental health.

The collective healing that transpires within the support group extends beyond individual recovery; it embodies a transformative process that empowers DeCola and his peers to reclaim their narratives and identities. Through shared vulnerability and support, DeCola finds not just healing but also a profound sense of empowerment and solidarity.

In essence, DeCola's participation in support groups, underscored by his embrace of vulnerability, becomes a pivotal element of his mental health recovery. The sense of community, shared healing, and collective wisdom gained from these groups enriches DeCola's journey, offering him a supportive network that underpins his path to well-being.

DeCola Learns from Others

DeCola's journey toward mental health recovery is significantly enhanced by his openness to learning from the experiences and coping strategies of others. This willingness to absorb and apply the wisdom of those who have navigated similar paths becomes a critical element of his healing process, enriching his approach to overcoming challenges.

Through interactions within support groups, therapy sessions, and even casual conversations, DeCola encounters a diverse array of perspectives and strategies for managing mental health. Each person's story offers unique insights into resilience, adaptability, and the nuanced ways in which individuals confront and cope with their struggles. For DeCola, these narratives become a rich source of learning, providing him with an expanded toolkit of coping mechanisms that he can tailor to his own needs.

Moreover, DeCola's openness facilitates a two-way exchange, where not only does he gain insights from others, but he also shares his own experiences, contributing to the collective pool of knowledge. This reciprocal exchange fosters a dynamic environment of mutual support and learning, where everyone's journey serves to inform and inspire others.

The coping strategies and insights DeCola learns from others are not limited to direct management of mental health symptoms. They also encompass broader life skills such as communication, boundary setting, and self-care practices that extend beyond mental health into overall well-being. By integrating these strategies into his daily life, DeCola enhances his resilience, emotional intelligence, and capacity for self-care, all of which are essential components of a sustainable recovery.

Furthermore, learning from others helps DeCola to cultivate empathy and understanding, both for himself and for those around him. Witnessing the diverse ways in which people cope with challenges broadens his perspective, fostering a more compassionate and non-judgmental approach to mental health. This expanded worldview not only aids in

DeCola's recovery but also enhances his relationships and interactions with others.

In essence, DeCola's openness to learning from the experiences and coping strategies of others is a cornerstone of his mental health recovery. This exchange of knowledge and support enriches his understanding of mental health, equipping him with a broad array of tools and perspectives that bolster his journey toward well-being. Through this process of shared learning, DeCola not only advances his recovery but also contributes to a culture of empathy, support, and collective growth within the mental health community.

DeCola Enhances Emotional Expression

DeCola's journey through mental health recovery is deeply enriched by his embrace of vulnerability, which unlocks a new realm of emotional expression for him. This newfound ability to articulate and navigate a wide spectrum of emotions with authenticity and depth marks a significant milestone in his healing journey, contributing to both his personal growth and overall well-being.

As DeCola opens himself up to vulnerability, he finds that the walls he had built around his emotions begin to crumble, allowing him to access and express feelings that were previously muted or ignored. This emotional awakening enables him to articulate feelings of joy, sadness, fear, and hope with greater clarity and intensity. By giving voice to these emotions, DeCola not only alleviates the burden of unspoken feelings but also fosters a deeper connection with his inner landscape, as well as with the people around him.

This enriched emotional expressiveness facilitates more meaningful interactions with friends, family, and even acquaintances. DeCola's ability to share his emotions openly invites others to respond in kind, leading to conversations and connections that are rooted in authenticity and mutual understanding. These interactions, built on the foundation of genuine emotional exchange, strengthen his support network and provide a sense of shared human experience.

Moreover, DeCola's enhanced emotional expression plays a crucial role in his therapeutic journey. In the safe space of therapy, his willingness to explore and articulate his emotions leads to profound insights and breakthroughs. This openness enables his therapist to tailor interventions more effectively, addressing the root causes of DeCola's struggles and facilitating a more impactful healing process.

The practice of expressing emotions also contributes to DeCola's resilience. By becoming comfortable with a wide range of emotions, he learns to navigate life's ups and downs with greater ease. This emotional agility allows him to face challenges without being overwhelmed, as he understands that emotions, no matter how intense, are transient and can be managed through expression and self-care.

Furthermore, DeCola's journey toward emotional expressiveness fosters a greater sense of self-acceptance and compassion. Recognizing that emotions are an integral part of the human experience, he learns to embrace his feelings without judgment, treating himself with the same kindness and understanding he offers others. This self-compassion reinforces his mental health recovery, providing a nurturing internal environment conducive to healing and growth.

In essence, DeCola's embrace of vulnerability and the resulting enhancement of his emotional expression is pivotal to his mental health recovery. This openness to experiencing and sharing a broad spectrum of emotions enriches his personal growth, strengthens his relationships, and forms a vital component of his journey toward healing and well-being. Through the power of vulnerability, DeCola discovers the transformative potential of emotional expressiveness, which becomes a key instrument in his recovery and a source of resilience in the face of life's challenges.

DeCola Shares His Story

As DeCola progresses on his path to mental health recovery, he begins to embrace the act of sharing his story with others, a step that holds profound implications for his healing process. This evolution from reticence to openness represents a significant breakthrough, as it involves overcoming the deeply ingrained fears of judgment and misunderstanding that often accompany discussions of mental health.

The act of sharing his journey serves as a cathartic release for DeCola, allowing him to externalize his experiences and emotions, which, until this point, may have been internalized and borne in silence. This verbalization of his struggles and triumphs transforms his narrative from a solitary burden into a shared experience, lightening the emotional load he carries and offering him a sense of liberation and relief.

Moreover, DeCola's willingness to articulate his journey creates a bridge of empathy and understanding with others who might be navigating their mental health challenges. His story becomes a beacon of hope and solidarity, sending a powerful message that no one is alone in their struggles. For those who hear his story, DeCola's experiences can validate their feelings, offer new perspectives, and perhaps most importantly, inspire courage to face their challenges.

Sharing his narrative also cultivates a deeper sense of community and belonging for DeCola. As he connects with others through the commonality of their experiences, he finds himself woven into a fabric of mutual support and understanding. This sense of being part of a larger community not only bolsters his resilience but also contributes to the collective strength of those connected by their shared journeys.

Furthermore, DeCola's openness invites dialogue and education, challenging misconceptions and stigmas surrounding mental health. Each time he shares his story, he chips away at the societal barriers that often silence discussions on mental well-being, fostering a more inclusive and compassionate environment.

In essence, DeCola's journey toward sharing his story is a testament to the healing power of vulnerability and connection. By moving beyond the fear of judgment and opening up about his experiences, DeCola not only advances his recovery but also contributes to a broader cultural shift towards openness, understanding, and support in the realm of mental health. Through this act of courage, he transforms his narrative from a personal odyssey into a shared journey of hope and resilience.

DeCola Practices Self-compassion

DeCola's embrace of vulnerability marks a pivotal turn in his mental health recovery, steering him toward the nurturing practice of self-compassion. This journey towards self-compassion is transformative, allowing DeCola to extend to himself the same kindness, patience, and understanding that he readily offers to others. This fundamental shift in how he relates to himself becomes a critical element of his healing process, fostering a healthier and more supportive internal environment.

As DeCola learns to be vulnerable and acknowledge his struggles openly, he confronts the often harsh and critical inner voice that had previously dictated his self-worth and his responses to challenges. Recognizing the destructive nature of self-criticism, he begins to cultivate a more compassionate inner dialogue. This new, kinder voice acknowledges his efforts, forgives his mistakes, and encourages him with empathy and understanding, much like a trusted friend would.

This practice of self-compassion encourages DeCola to view his experiences, especially setbacks and failures, through a lens of kindness and learning rather than judgment and defeat. He comes to understand that imperfections and vulnerabilities are inherent aspects of the human experience, not indications of personal failure. This perspective shift helps DeCola to accept and embrace his whole self, including his flaws and challenges, fostering a sense of wholeness and self-acceptance.

Furthermore, self-compassion becomes a source of resilience for DeCola, offering him a buffer against the inevitable stresses and adversities of life. By treating himself compassionately, he is better equipped to navigate difficult emotions and situations without being overwhelmed. This resilience allows him to face challenges with a sense of confidence and stability, knowing that he can rely on his inner kindness to support him through tough times.

Self-compassion also enhances DeCola's emotional well-being by promoting a more balanced approach to self-care. Recognizing the importance of nurturing his mental, physical, and emotional health, he prioritizes activities and practices that support his well-being. This holistic approach to self-care, grounded in self-compassion, ensures that De-Cola's recovery is sustainable and integrated into his daily life.

In essence, DeCola's development of self-compassion through embracing vulnerability is a cornerstone of his mental health recovery. This nurturing practice reshapes his relationship with himself, fostering an internal environment of kindness, forgiveness, and understanding. As DeCola cultivates self-compassion, he not only accelerates his healing but also builds a foundation for lasting well-being and resilience.

DeCola Inspires Others

DeCola's mental health recovery journey, characterized by his courage to embrace and share his vulnerabilities openly, transcends his healing to become a source of inspiration for others. His willingness to unveil the intricacies of his struggles and the steps he takes toward recovery resonate deeply within his community, sparking a transformative ripple effect that fosters a broader culture of openness, healing, and mutual support.

As DeCola shares his story, he becomes a living testament to the strength inherent in vulnerability. His narrative, replete with challenges, setbacks, and triumphs, serves as a beacon of hope for those who may feel isolated or overwhelmed by their mental health struggles. Witnessing DeCola's journey, others are encouraged to reconsider their perspectives on vulnerability, recognizing it not as a weakness but as a courageous step toward self-awareness and healing.

DeCola's openness acts as a catalyst, breaking down the barriers of silence and stigma that often surround mental health issues. By speaking candidly about his experiences, he creates a safe space for dialogue where others feel empowered to share their stories. This collective sharing fosters a sense of solidarity and understanding within the community, making it clear that no one has to navigate their mental health journey alone.

Furthermore, DeCola's story highlights the importance of seeking help and utilizing available support systems, from therapy and support groups to community resources. His proactive approach to recovery demystifies the process of seeking assistance, encouraging others to explore and embrace the support options available to them. This shift towards active engagement with mental health care contributes to a community-wide increase in mental well-being and re-silience.

The ripple effect of DeCola's journey extends beyond individual inspiration, contributing to a cultural shift within his community. As more individuals feel inspired to embrace their vulnerabilities and seek support, the collective narrative around mental health begins to change. This evolving narrative fosters a more inclusive, empathetic, and supportive environment where mental health is prioritized, and individuals feel valued and understood.

In essence, DeCola's journey and his decision to share it openly become a powerful force for change, inspiring others to embrace their vulnerabilities and seek the support they need. His story not only contributes to his recovery but also ignites a ripple effect of healing, support, and transformation within his community, showcasing the profound impact one individual's journey can have on collective well-being.

DeCola Fosters Growth

DeCola's journey through mental health recovery, characterized by an embrace of vulnerability, becomes a powerful catalyst for profound personal growth. This transformative process enables him to navigate through and beyond the realm of his fears, facilitating a deeper understanding of his identity and enriching his engagement with life and relationships.

By allowing himself to be vulnerable, DeCola confronts his fears head-on rather than avoiding or masking them. This confrontation is not merely a battle but a process of understanding the roots of his fears, acknowledging their presence, and gradually learning to diminish their control over his life. Each fear confronted marks a step towards liberation, opening up new avenues for exploration and experience that were previously hindered by apprehension and self-doubt.

This journey of facing fears is closely tied to the evolution of DeCola's identity. Vulnerability peels back the layers of persona built up over time, revealing the authentic self beneath. This revelation is not without its challenges, as it demands that DeCola reconcile the various facets of his being—both the strengths and the vulnerabilities. However, through this reconciliation, he discovers a more cohesive and authentic sense of self. This newfound self-awareness grants him the freedom to redefine his values, aspirations, and the paths he chooses to pursue, aligning them more closely with his true self.

Furthermore, DeCola's embrace of vulnerability significantly enhances the quality of his relationships. By being open and authentic, he invites a similar level of depth and sincerity from others. This mutual vulnerability fosters deeper connections built on a foundation of trust, empathy, and genuine understanding. Relationships become more meaningful, providing not only support and companionship but also opportunities for mutual growth and enrichment.

DeCola's vulnerability also opens up a broader spectrum of emotional experience, allowing him to engage more fully with life's highs and lows. This emotional richness adds depth to his experiences, making moments of joy more vibrant and instances of sorrow more profound yet manageable. This heightened emotional engagement brings a greater sense of fulfillment and presence to DeCola's life pursuits, whether in personal projects, hobbies, or professional endeavors.

In essence, DeCola's embrace of vulnerability acts as a springboard for significant personal growth. It challenges him to confront and move beyond his fears, fosters a more authentic identity, enriches his relationships, and deepens his engagement with life. This transformative journey not only propels DeCola's mental health recovery forward but also elevates his overall experience of life, imbuing it with a sense of purpose, connection, and fulfillment.

In embracing vulnerability, DeCola not only advances his mental health recovery but also contributes to a cultural shift towards greater openness, compassion, and collective support for mental well-being.

Chapter 6: The Journey Through Therapy

DeCola's journey towards recovery amidst the tangled web of mental health challenges was a witness to the enduring spirit of human resilience. Appointments, crucial lifelines in the vast sea of turmoil, often felt like distant, shimmering mirages on the horizon. They were elusive, seemingly always just out of reach, compounding DeCola's sense of isolation in his struggle. The professionals he encountered along the way, though well-intentioned and immersed in their craft, sometimes seemed to speak in a dialect foreign to DeCola's immediate needs. Their meticulous approach, while admirable, occasionally felt dragged against the chaotic backdrop of DeCola's inner turmoil. Their words, meant to heal, at times, felt like echoes in a void, unable to bridge the chasm to DeCola's silent scream of suffering.

This journey, marked by its share of setbacks, served as a poignant reminders of the intricate complexities woven into the very fabric of seeking mental health support. Each stumbling block, each bureaucratic hurdle, cast long, daunting shadows over DeCola's path to healing. These obstacles were not mere inconveniences but towering monuments to the systemic challenges entrenched within the pursuit of mental well-being.

Society's echo chamber, with its subtle and not-so-subtle stigmas surrounding mental health, often seemed to amplify DeCola's internal fears. The pervasive notion that seeking help equated to a lack of personal strength rather than an act of courage added layers of internal conflict to his battle. It was a struggle not just against his mind but against the societal constructs that shaped his perception of strength and vulnerability.

Yet, within this blend of challenges, the smoldering hope within DeCola refused to be extinguished. It flickered, resilient against the blasts of despair, a testament to the indomitable spirit that had driven him to seek help in the first place. This hope, though at times feeble and wavering, was the silent beacon guiding him through the darkest nights of his soul.

This chapter of DeCola's life, fraught with the rawness of awakening to his vulnerabilities and the convoluted path to aid, laid the foundational stones for a transformative journey. It was a journey that would meander through the shadowed valleys of despair and the luminous peaks of enlightenment, a journey symbolic of rediscovery, resilience, and unyielding resolve.

As DeCola traversed this landscape of healing, he found himself rekindling the vibrancy of life that seemed forever captured in the reddish, brown-toned photographs of yesteryears. Each step forward, each moment of connection with his therapists, and each breakthrough in understanding his psyche wove a tapestry of recovery that was uniquely his. This journey was not just about reclaiming the life once depicted in photographs but about reimagining a future where the echoes of past sufferings transformed into the harmonies of healing and hope.

In the monotony of an ordinary day, a moment of coincidence transformed DeCola's life. It was a chance encounter with an old friend, a figure who had quietly drifted to the periphery of DeCola's world. This friend, bearing the marks of his battles with mental health, shared stories of struggle and triumph that resonated deeply with DeCola. Their rekindled connection, warmed by genuine empathy and understanding, became a reflective surface for DeCola's own experiences. No longer were his struggles a solitary journey;

they were part of a shared human narrative, rich with the promise of healing.

This encounter, seemingly simple, ignited a spark within DeCola. It was the dawning realization that he was not isolated in his struggles; the shadows he fought had names, faces, and stories like his own. The exchange of vulnerabilities and acts of courage between DeCola and his friend served as a catalyst, jolting him into a newfound awareness of his condition. What once was shrouded in denial slowly began to take shape as a reality he could no longer ignore.

Fuelled by the resilience he saw mirrored in his friend and a budding sense of optimism, DeCola made a pivotal choice to embrace change. Despite the trepidation that shadowed this decision, it marked the first step towards a journey of recovery. The path was fraught with challenges, from navigating the complex mental health care system to confronting societal stigmas. Yet, DeCola's resolve, fortified by the knowledge that he was not alone, propelled him forward.

As DeCola stepped into the world of therapy, he encountered an environment vastly different from the turbulent seas of his struggles. Each therapist's office, a sanctuary lined with volumes of scientific innovations or psychological wisdom, became the backdrop for his transformative journey. Initially, therapy sessions oscillated between dialogue and contemplation, challenging DeCola to articulate thoughts and emotions long silenced. The therapeutic path was a fusion of moments—some illuminating, others daunting—each uniquely tailored to unravel the intricate web of DeCola's psyche.

At the core of DeCola's healing was the evolving partnership with his therapists. This unique bond, built on the bedrock of vulnerability and trust, became DeCola's steadfast anchor. In the therapist's empathetic reflection, DeCola saw not only the depths of his despair but also the flickers of potential and hope within himself.

Thus, DeCola keeps striving to traverse an undulating path of the highs and lows, where light often springs from the depths of darkness. Each step was a beat in the rhythm of resilience, with dazzling insights breaking through the heavy clouds of challenge. He moved with the grace of a dancer through the complex choreography of recovery, crafting a story that paid tribute to his history even as it etched a trail to a rejuvenated tomorrow. In this way, DeCola set forth on a metamorphic expedition, its destination shaping itself with every twist and turn of the path.

This narrative intricately weaves DeCola's therapeutic recovery, underpinned by the concerted efforts of dedicated professionals from various disciplines. Their collaboration forms the cornerstone of DeCola's healing, transcending the conventional approach to therapy. It's not about quick fixes or miraculous recoveries; it's about embarking on a sacred expedition of self-discovery, growth, and profound transformation.

Through DeCola's lens, we are privy to the delicate yet powerful unfolding of his healing process. It's a path characterized by the rawness of vulnerability and the sheer courage to confront one's shadows. DeCola's journey is a testament to the human spirit's resilience, an inspiring narrative that underscores the importance of hope as an eternal flame, illuminating the darkest corners of despair and guiding him toward a dawn of renewed possibility.

As DeCola navigates this complex landscape of mental health recovery, each therapeutic session becomes a chapter in his larger story of rebirth. These encounters with therapists are not mere conversations but are transformative experiences that challenge him to peel away the layers of his pain and confront the core of his struggles. It's within these sacred spaces of therapy rooms that DeCola learns more about the art of resilience, the power of introspection, and the beauty of emotional liberation.

"Subscribed to Live" beautifully encapsulates the essence of DeCola's healing journey, portraying it as a mosaic of human experiences. It's a narrative that celebrates the triumphs and acknowledges the setbacks, painting a realistic picture of what it means to journey through therapy. It's a story that resonates with anyone who has ever dared to seek help, to change, and to believe in the possibility of a brighter future.

In this journey, DeCola emerges not just as a participant in his therapy but as an active architect of his recovery. Each step forward, each insight gained, and each moment of connection with his therapists contribute to a larger picture of healing. It's a process that fosters a deep understanding of oneself, an awakening to the inherent strength within, and an unwavering commitment to forge a path toward wellness.

"Subscribed to Thrive: A Mental Health Resolve" is thus a poignant reminder of the transformative power of therapy, seen through the eyes of DeCola. It is a silent witness to his evolution. It's a narrative that intertwines vulnerability, courage, and hope, offering a ray of light to those embarking on their journey of recovery.

The Overview of DeCola's Therapy Plan

DeCola's journey through his challenges was akin to following a map drawn up with care and understanding, each step placed with his well-being in mind. From the outset, it was clear that this path was crafted uniquely for him, with every twist and turn tailored to guide him back to a place where life felt more manageable.

It all started with a gathering that put DeCola at the heart of the conversation, surrounded by those he trusted. Together, they mapped out a route that felt right for him, infused with the collective wisdom of his guides and the unwavering support of his loved ones. This plan was distinctly DeCola's, respecting his preferences and needs at every juncture.

A pivotal moment for DeCola was forming a connection with someone who truly understood the terrain he was navigating. This relationship wasn't about following a predetermined path; it was about discovering the pathways that resonated with DeCola, whether it was unpacking his thoughts or finding new strategies to face his obstacles head-on.

The support from his family and friends wasn't just about their presence; it was about them being there in a way that bolstered DeCola, ensuring they were pillars of support rather than added pressures.

When DeCola's path involved medication, the focus was on mindful monitoring, ensuring the benefits outweighed any concerns. Open conversations about his feelings towards medication kept DeCola aligned with his care approach, ensuring he remained in harmony with the chosen strategies.

Incorporating the rhythms of daily life was also crucial, emphasizing the importance of activity, nutrition, and rest, all tailored to fit seamlessly into DeCola's life, enhancing his overall well-being.

The strategy laid out for DeCola was flexible, adapting to his evolving needs and ensuring that the support he required was always within reach, whether it was a one-on-one talk or the camaraderie of a group.

Understanding his journey better, both for DeCola and his circle, demystified his experience, laying a foundation for hopeful, realistic progress and a mutual comprehension of the way forward.

DeCola's story indicates how a journey through crisis doesn't just hinge on one thing; it's about weaving together everything that matters to the person at the heart of it all, making sure the path forward is as clear and as comfortable as it can be for them and those they share their life with.

In DeCola's journey through a particularly tough time with his mental health, his path to feeling better was paved with a plan that looked at him as a whole person, not just the problems he was facing. This plan was like a tapestry, woven with different strands that together aimed to bring him back to a place of strength and stability.

At the heart of DeCola's journey was the support he got from trained personnel who really understood the kind of challenges he was up against. This wasn't just about sitting and talking; it was about finding the right ways for DeCola to work through what he was feeling, to learn new ways to handle tough moments, and to make sense of the deeper issues that were weighing on him. These regular heart-to-hearts gave DeCola a safe space to open up and start piecing things back together.

Part of finding his way through the storm involved learning how to stand firm when things got really rough. DeCola picked up some handy tricks to keep his feet on the ground, like ways to pull his thoughts back to the present moment and quick fixes for when the pressure seemed too much.

The world around DeCola played a big part, too. Finding a community that got what he was going through made a world of difference. It was like finding a group of fellow travelers on a similar journey, offering each other nods of understanding and sharing what worked for them. And then there was his circle of family and friends, who, once they got the lowdown on how best to be there for DeCola, became an even stronger network of support, making his day-to-day world a more understanding place.

Whenever DeCola's path included medication, navigating this part was all about finding a balance that felt right for him, with someone keeping a close eye to make sure it was helping more than hurting. Talking openly about how he felt about taking medication and finding something that fits without too many downsides was key.

DeCola's story really highlights how a thoughtful, kind-hearted approach to getting through a mental health crisis can make all the difference. By piecing together a plan step by step, tailored just for him, it wasn't just about getting through the tough times; it was about recognizing DeCola's full humanity, his strengths, and his potential to find his way back to solid ground.

From the very start, DeCola's journey to feeling better began with getting to know him, really digging deep to understand what he was going through. This wasn't just about ticking boxes or filling out forms; it was about building a connection based on real trust and understanding. This personal touch meant that every step of the plan made for De-Cola felt like it was truly his, giving him a real stake in his journey forward.

As things moved forward, it wasn't just one person by DeCola's side but a whole team, each bringing their special skills to the table. They looked at everything that mattered to DeCola's well-being, from how he was feeling inside to how he was taking care of his body, who he had around him, and so much more. This team effort was all about seeing the big picture, making sure DeCola had all-round support.

The moment when improvement was becoming apparent was in the aftermath, as DeCola noticed the positive changes from all the hard work. It was a time to reflect, to plan for the days ahead, and to slowly ease back into the flow of everyday life with new skills and confidence. This part of the journey was all about building on the progress made, laying down solid groundwork for a future where DeCola felt strong and ready for whatever came his way.

But it didn't just stop there; DeCola knew he had an ongoing circle of support. Regular check-ins and tweaks to his plan meant that as his life changed, so too could the support around him, keeping him feeling secure and confident in his ability to keep up his well-being.

DeCola's story is a testament to the power of a well-rounded, caring approach when facing tough times. It's about more than just getting through a crisis; it's about learning, growing, and finding hope again. With a careful plan and a team ready to support him at every turn, DeCola's journey was about paving a path to recovery filled with resilience, growth, and a brighter outlook for the future.

As DeCola embarked on his therapeutic journey, guided by a team of multidisciplinary professionals, he began to witness a profound transformation within himself. This wasn't a sudden change but a gradual unfolding, like the slow blooming of a flower at the first hint of spring. Each session, each conversation, was a step towards reclaiming the vitality and peace that mental illness had shadowed.

Initially, the progress was subtle, almost invisible. Yet, DeCola remained committed, trusting in the process and the expertise of his therapists. They worked together, weaving a tapestry of traditional and innovative therapies tailored specifically to his needs. This bespoke approach ensured that each aspect of his well-being was addressed, from the cognitive distortions that clouded his mind to the emotional turmoil that weighed heavily on his heart.

As the weeks turned into months, the changes became more pronounced. The heavy fog of anxiety that had once seemed impenetrable began to lift, revealing clearer skies ahead. The depressive episodes that had anchored him in darkness became less frequent and less intense, allowing rays of hope and joy to filter through. It was as if DeCola was emerging from a long, arduous winter into the rejuvenating warmth of spring.

The therapy sessions, once daunting, became sources of strength and enlightenment. DeCola learned strategies to navigate his thoughts and emotions, tools that empowered him to face life's challenges with resilience and grace. He discovered the healing power of articulating his fears and dreams, of unraveling the complex web of his psyche in a safe and supportive environment.

This journey was not without its challenges, for healing is rarely a linear path. There were days when old patterns resurfaced, threatening to undo the progress he had made. But DeCola, bolstered by the unwavering support of his therapists and the inner strength he had cultivated, faced these setbacks with courage. Each hurdle surmounted added a new layer of confidence and self-awareness, fortifying his journey towards wellness.

As DeCola continued to traverse the therapeutic path, the transformation within him became undeniable. The symptoms of his mental illness, once a constant presence, gradually receded into the background, losing their grip on his life. He found himself reconnecting with his passions, engaging more fully with the world around him, and forging deeper, more meaningful relationships.

In this gradual yet profound process, DeCola rediscovered his healthy self, not merely returning to who he was before but emerging stronger, more resilient, and more attuned to the beauty and complexity of life. This journey through therapy, marked by incremental healing and personal growth, illuminated the path to a brighter, healthier future.

DeCola and the Therapists

DeCola understood and agreed that his sessions with various professionals would be coordinated yet spaced out to avoid overwhelming him. He knew he could reschedule if necessary and that there might be some overlap in their approaches. This repetition was explained as a way to reinforce different facets of his recovery, each from a unique professional perspective.

As DeCola progresses through his therapy journey, it's important to note that his treatment involves a network of specialists, each contributing their unique expertise to his care. However, this narrative does not encompass the full spectrum of professionals and additional referrals that play a role in his recovery. The focus here is on a select few whose interventions are critical and illustrative of the broader therapeutic process, providing a glimpse into the collaborative effort behind his path to wellness. This approach allows for a deeper exploration of certain therapeutic relationships and techniques, shedding light on their significance in DeCola's journey while acknowledging the existence of other influential figures and practices beyond the scope of this account.

DeCola and His Doctor (GP)

In the tapestry of DeCola's recovery journey, the threads of professional guidance and personal dedication intertwine, with his General Practitioner (GP) playing an instrumental role. The story begins with a pivotal meeting where DeCola, bearing the weight of his mental health struggles, seeks refuge in the expertise of his GP. This initial consultation unfolds as a deep dive into DeCola's life, a conversation that traverses the landscape of his emotions, daily routines, and the stressors that shadow his existence. This dialogue, rich in detail and empathy, provides the GP with a comprehensive portrait of DeCola's mental health landscape.

Recognizing the need for specialized care, the GP becomes the architect of the next phase in DeCola's journey, steering him toward a mental health specialist renowned for their expertise. This referral is not merely administrative; it is a thoughtful recommendation tailored to DeCola's unique circumstances, considering his preferences and the specific challenges he faces.

Embarking on this new chapter, DeCola meets with the specialist, where he undergoes an extensive evaluation. This process, intricate and nuanced, employs a spectrum of diagnostic tools to unravel the complexities of DeCola's mental health. It is a journey into the depths of his psyche, aimed at unearthing the roots of his distress.

With a roadmap of DeCola's mental landscape in hand, a personalized treatment plan begins to take shape. This bespoke blueprint for recovery encompasses a series of therapeutic approaches, with what is termed 'Cognitive Behavioral Therapy (CBT)' taking center stage. It's a collaborative effort, one that includes medication under the vigilant oversight of his GP, lifestyle adjustments, and a network of support tailored to DeCola's evolving needs.

As DeCola navigates the healing process through therapy sessions, the synergy between him, his leading specialist, and his GP forms the bedrock of his journey. This triad of trust ensures a holistic approach to DeCola's well-being, especially when navigating the complexities of medication and the interconnections between physical and mental health.

DeCola's journey is marked by continuous evolution, with his treatment plan undergoing regular reassessment to mirror his feedback and shifting needs. It's a dynamic, collaborative process, with DeCola at its heart, seamlessly integrated by his GP and the specialist.

Recovery, however, is not the destination. The organization chosen by DeCola for support transitions into a role of ongoing guardianship and offers maintenance sessions to fortify DeCola's mental health in the long term.

When the time comes to celebrate the milestones of recovery, DeCola's therapy journey reaches a thoughtful conclusion. Armed with the tools and strategies forged through his experiences and the wisdom to seek support when needed, DeCola stands ready to navigate the ebb and flow of life's challenges. This journey, underscored by the steadfast support of his GP and the leading specialist, embodies the essence of a personalized pathway to healing and hope.

DeCola and His Psychiatrist

DeCola's therapy journey towards recovery is significantly enhanced by the specialized involvement of a social psychiatrist, whose expertise lies in understanding the complex interplay between social environments and mental health. This unique partnership begins with an insightful consultation, where DeCola and the psychiatrist delve into the depth of DeCola's life, exploring his social circles, relationships, and past experiences. This conversation is not merely clinical; it is an empathetic exploration aimed at painting a full picture of DeCola's world, both internal and external.

Following this initial meeting, a more comprehensive evaluation, generally described as a 'biopsychosocial' assessment, is conducted, weaving together the biological, physical, psychological, and social strands that define DeCola's current mental state. This assessment is pivotal, as it lays the foundation for a treatment plan that is not only attuned to DeCola's immediate mental health needs but also mindful of the broader social and environmental factors that influence his well-being.

As the journey unfolds, DeCola is introduced to what the psychiatrist called 'psychotherapy' sessions. These sessions are meticulously designed to enhance DeCola's coping mechanisms and resilience in the face of life's inevitable stressors. Where necessary, medication management is impeccably incorporated into his care, ensuring a holistic approach to his mental health challenges.

Recognizing the indispensable role of social connections in DeCola's recovery, the social psychiatrist guides him in fortifying his support networks. This aspect of the treatment acknowledges the therapeutic power of community and the strength found in meaningful relationships. DeCola is encouraged to engage with his community, fostering connections that offer support and understanding, thereby reinforcing his mental health recovery framework.

The dynamic nature of DeCola's recovery journey is maintained through regular check-ins and the flexibility to adjust his treatment plan as needed. This adaptable approach ensures that his pathway to recovery is always aligned with his progressive needs, embodying a truly personalized care treatment.

As DeCola makes strides in his recovery, the emphasis of his therapy gradually shifts towards maintenance and relapse prevention. The social psychiatrist remains a pillar of support, offering ongoing guidance to sustain the progress DeCola has achieved. This enduring partnership equips De-Cola with the confidence and skills to maintain his mental health even as he faces future challenges.

This comprehensive and meticulous approach, deeply rooted in an understanding of the social dimensions of mental health, empowers DeCola to embark on his recovery journey with a robust support system. It provides him with a set of tools and strategies tailored to navigate the complexities of mental health, ensuring a resilient foundation for his continued well-being.

DeCola and His General Psychologist

In DeCola's journey to overcome a mental health crisis, collaborating with a social psychologist becomes a significant chapter, focusing on the intricate ways social dynamics influence his well-being. The partnership begins with a comprehensive exploration of DeCola's social world, discussing how interactions, societal expectations, and community ties shape his mental health landscape.

Together, they pinpoint the social elements at play—be it the strength of DeCola's support network, societal pressures he faces, or the nuances of his interpersonal relationships. They delve into how these factors either serve as pillars of support or sources of stress, unraveling the complex interplay between social environment and mental well-being.

The exploration extends to DeCola's social cognition—how he perceives, interprets, and reacts within his social sphere. This might involve dissecting situations that trigger discomfort or examining the underlying assumptions guiding his social perceptions.

To navigate the social labyrinth more adeptly, DeCola and the psychologist co-develop a suite of social strategies. This ranged from honing communication skills to mastering conflict resolution, all aimed at enriching DeCola's social engagements.

Addressing cognitive and social biases forms another cornerstone of their work, challenging prejudiced perceptions that might color DeCola's social experiences negatively. By reshaping these perceptions, they pave the way for more balanced and positive social interactions.

Strengthening DeCola's social fabric is crucial, fortifying existing bonds and weaving new ones, thereby enriching his support system. This process not only nurtures DeCola's relationships but also deepens his sense of belonging within his social circles.

The psychologist guides DeCola in aligning more closely with communities and groups that reflect his values and interests, bolstering his social identity and fostering a deeper sense of connection.

DeCola immersed himself in social psychological interventions, such as participating in group therapies or community initiatives, which further cement his understanding of social dynamics and their impact on his mental health.

Regular check-ins allow DeCola and the psychologist to gauge progress and adapt strategies to the evolving social landscape, ensuring that DeCola's growth remains responsive to his changing needs and circumstances.

Ultimately, the aim is for DeCola to stand confidently within his social world, equipped with the skills and insights to maintain his mental health autonomously. This gradual transition is marked by the development of a personal blueprint for ongoing social engagement and mental health management, a testament to the transformative power of understanding and navigating the social dimensions of mental well-being.

DeCola and His Neuropsychologist

DeCola's path to mental health recovery takes a significant turn when he begins working with a neuropsychologist, focusing on the critical link between his brain function and psychological experiences. This partnership kicks off with an in-depth analysis of DeCola's cognitive and emotional landscape, considering how his brain's workings influence his thoughts, feelings, and behavior.

The collaboration involves identifying key neurological factors that might be affecting DeCola's mental health. This encompasses exploration of the impact of genes inherited, any brain injuries, neurological conditions, or simply the way DeCola's brain processes information and emotions. They delve into the science of nerve cells underlying his mental health challenges, unraveling how biological factors interplay with his psychological state.

As they uncover how DeCola's brain influences his perception and interaction with the world, they tailor cognitive and behavioral strategies to navigate these challenges more effectively. This includes cognitive rehabilitation exercises, strategies to enhance memory and attention, or techniques to manage emotional responses more effectively.

Addressing potential barriers to brain functions, such as difficulties with attention, memory, or executive functioning, becomes a core focus. By tackling these issues, DeCola experiences more positive interactions and a greater sense of control over his thoughts and actions.

Boosting DeCola's cognitive foundations is crucial, potentially involving exercises to enhance brain function or strategies to compensate for any anomalies. This approach not only enhances DeCola's cognitive skills but also builds resilience against future psychological stress.

The neuropsychologist also helps DeCola integrate his cognitive strategies with his everyday life, ensuring that he can apply what he's learned in real-world situations. This involved practical applications of memory aids, mindfulness techniques, or customized strategies to improve problem-solving and decision-making.

Regular sessions provide a space for DeCola and the neuropsychologist to assess progress and refine strategies, ensuring that the approach evolves with DeCola's ongoing needs and the latest neuropsychological insights.

The goal is for DeCola to achieve a level of cognitive and emotional autonomy, equipped with a deep understanding of how his brain functions and how he can leverage this knowledge to maintain his mental health. This journey culminates in DeCola developing a personal plan that incorporates neuropsychological principles into his daily life, empowering him to navigate his world with confidence and resilience, grounded in a better understanding of the neurological applications underpinning his mental well-being.

DeCola and His Psychiatric Nurses

DeCola's road to mental health recovery is significantly supported by the dedicated involvement of mental health nurses, who provide a multifaceted layer of care tailored to his unique needs. The journey begins with an in-depth evaluation by the nurse, who meticulously gathers insights into

DeCola's mental and physical health history, current treatment regimen, and lifestyle, laying the groundwork for a customized care approach.

From this foundational assessment, a collaborative care plan emerges, crafted with DeCola's active input and, where suitable, his family's. This plan sets clear recovery objectives and outlines the nursing interventions poised to guide De-Cola toward his goals alongside metrics to track progress.

Medication management becomes a cornerstone of De-Cola's care, with the nurse meticulously overseeing the administration of treatments, monitoring their impact, and educating DeCola about their purposes and expected benefits, all while vigilantly managing any side effects.

The nurse also engages DeCola in therapeutic conversations, offering a blend of emotional support, empathy, and active listening to foster a trust-based therapeutic alliance essential for DeCola's recovery journey.

Education extends beyond medication to encompass a broad spectrum of coping mechanisms, stress management techniques, and lifestyle modifications conducive to mental health recovery. This educational outreach covers areas such as exercise, dietary habits, sleep routines, and relaxation practices.

DeCola benefits from continuous support and monitoring, with the nurse regularly evaluating his mental health status and treatment responses to ensure the care plan remains dynamic and responsive to his evolving needs.

The nurse plays a fundamental role in coordinating DeCola's multidisciplinary care, ensuring seamless collaboration across his healthcare team, which includes psychiatrists, therapists, and other specialists, to maintain a unified approach to his recovery.

Crisis intervention capabilities are an integral part of the nurse's role, providing immediate support to stabilize DeCola's condition during acute episodes, reassess treatment strategies, and connect him with additional resources as needed.

Promoting social connectivity and community involvement forms part of DeCola's recovery strategy, with the nurse encouraging participation in activities and groups that foster a sense of belonging and reinforce his support network.

As DeCola progresses, the nurse assists in planning for his transition to subsequent care phases or his return to daily life activities, focusing on sustainable recovery and the anticipation of potential challenges post-treatment.

Regular evaluations of the care plan's efficacy, conducted in partnership with DeCola and his broader care team, ensure that his treatment remains adaptable and fine-tuned to his changing needs and circumstances over time.

In this comprehensive care framework, the mental health nurse stands as a crucial ally, educator, and advocate, contributing profoundly to DeCola's holistic care and supporting his journey toward lasting mental health recovery.

DeCola and His Dietician

DeCola's incorporation of nutritional guidance into his mental health recovery strategy marks a significant step towards holistic well-being, with a dietitian playing a crucial role in this journey. Their collaboration commences with an in-depth discussion aimed at mapping out DeCola's existing dietary patterns, lifestyle choices, and their interplay with his mental health challenges. This initial dialogue sets the stage for a thorough nutritional assessment, pinpointing any dietary imbalances or deficiencies that could be influencing DeCola's psychological state.

Together, DeCola and the dietitian establish nutrition-related objectives designed to bolster his mental health recovery. These goals are carefully crafted to be both attainable and supportive of DeCola's well-being, with a focus on enhancing his mood, energy, and overall mental equilibrium.

A customized nutrition plan emerges from this collaborative effort, offering DeCola a roadmap to a diet that not only nourishes his body but also supports his mental health. This plan addresses key nutritional considerations and is complemented by practical meal preparation advice and strategies to navigate dietary challenges.

Education plays a central role in DeCola's journey, equipping him with knowledge about the profound connection between diet and mental well-being. He learns about brain-boosting foods, mood-stabilizing nutrients, and techniques to combat emotional eating, all integral to his path to recovery.

Ongoing support through regular check-ins with the dietitian ensures that DeCola's nutrition plan remains responsive to his needs, adjusting as necessary to reflect his progress and any new challenges he encounters. These sessions are vital for sustaining motivation and adapting the nutritional strategy to support his mental health journey best.

In an ideal scenario, DeCola's dietitian and mental health care providers work in harmony, fostering a cohesive treatment strategy that integrates nutritional and psychological support. This collaborative approach ensures that DeCola's dietary advancements are harmonized with his broader mental health objectives.

As DeCola progresses, the impact of his dietary changes on his mental health is continually assessed, with adjustments made to optimize outcomes. Celebrating milestones in his recovery reinforces the positive shifts in his well-being and encourages adherence to healthy eating habits.

The journey eventually transitions to a focus on long-term maintenance, with the dietitian guiding to help DeCola sustain the healthy dietary practices that have become a cornerstone of his mental health recovery. This ongoing support is adaptable and ready to evolve alongside DeCola's lifestyle and any new challenges he may face, ensuring that his nutritional well-being continues to support his mental health in the long run.

DeCola and His Physiotherapist

DeCola's path to mental health recovery is enriched by incorporating a structured physical activity regimen guided by a physiotherapist who specializes in marrying exercise with mental wellness. The collaboration kicks off with a detailed evaluation of DeCola's physical condition, his current activity level, and any specific health constraints, all viewed through the lens of his mental health journey.

This initial step lays the foundation for a dialogue about DeCola's exercise preferences and what he hopes to achieve through physical activity, whether it's stress alleviation, mood enhancement, or a boost in energy. This ensures the resulting exercise plan resonates with DeCola, incorporating activities he's genuinely interested in and motivated to pursue.

The physiotherapist then crafts an adapted exercise schedule tailored to DeCola's unique needs and recovery goals. This plan thoughtfully balances exercise types, intensities, and frequencies to support DeCola's mental health objectives while being mindful of his enjoyment and safety.

Education forms a crucial part of this process, with the physiotherapist illuminating the profound impact of physical activity on mental health. DeCola learns about the psychological and physiological benefits of exercise, from mood regulation to stress relief, empowering him with the knowledge to support his recovery journey.

The implementation of DeCola's exercise plan is gradual, allowing him to adapt comfortably and build confidence in his abilities. This phased approach helps foster a sustainable routine that DeCola can integrate effortlessly into his life.

Throughout this journey, the physiotherapist remains a steadfast source of encouragement, adapting the exercise regimen as needed and celebrating DeCola's milestones. This ongoing support is pivotal in helping DeCola navigate challenges and stay committed to his physical wellness goals.

Regular evaluations ensure the exercise plan remains aligned with DeCola's evolving needs and mental health status, with adjustments made to keep the activities effective and engaging.

Ideally, this physical wellness strategy is woven into DeCola's broader mental health care, creating a cohesive treatment approach. The physiotherapist and mental health professionals collaborate to ensure DeCola's physical activity complements his overall recovery plan.

As DeCola gains autonomy in his exercise routine, the physiotherapist equips him with the tools and knowledge to maintain his physical activity independently, ensuring he understands the long-term value of exercise for mental health.

The journey concludes with a reflective evaluation of the benefits DeCola has experienced from integrating exercise into his recovery, setting the stage for future fitness goals or maintaining the positive habits he has developed. This holistic approach underscores the critical role of physical activity in mental health recovery, offering DeCola a robust foundation for lasting well-being.

DeCola and His Social Worker

DeCola's engagement with a social worker marks a significant phase in his mental health recovery, where the focus is on navigating the intricate web of social, environmental, and psychological influences on his well-being. Social workers are adept at offering support, championing individuals' rights, and connecting them with essential resources to enhance DeCola's quality of life.

The journey commences with a thorough assessment by the social worker to gauge DeCola's mental health status, his interactions within social and family circles, his financial condition, living arrangements, and any other pertinent life facets. This comprehensive evaluation sheds light on the numerous factors that bear upon DeCola's mental health.

With the social worker's guidance, DeCola articulates his pressing needs and longer-term aspirations, which could span from securing necessities like shelter and nutrition to more complex objectives like mending family ties or rejoining the workforce.

From here, a tailor-made action plan emerges, crafted collaboratively by DeCola and the social worker. This blueprint delineates the measures necessary to cater to DeCola's requirements, harness his strengths, and realize his ambitions, blending immediate solutions with strategies for sustained progress.

The social worker then steers DeCola towards a spectrum of resources and services conducive to his recovery, such as mental health support, community groups, financial aid, educational opportunities, and healthcare provisions. Acting as an intermediary, the social worker facilitates DeCola's access to these supports, advocating on his behalf as needed.

An integral aspect of the social worker's role is equipping DeCola with essential life skills, thereby empowering him to manage his circumstances and advocate for his own needs effectively. This education covers problem-solving tactics, stress management, effective communication, and decision-making strategies.

Ongoing assistance and periodic evaluations are provided by the social worker, offering DeCola a stable support system. This continuous oversight allows for the fine-tuning of DeCola's action plan in response to his changing needs and life situations.

The social worker also collaborates with the broader team of professionals involved in DeCola's care, ensuring a cohesive and comprehensive treatment approach that addresses all facets of his well-being.

In advocating for DeCola, the social worker ensures his rights are upheld and his perspectives are recognized across various platforms, including healthcare, legal, and social service arenas.

Moreover, the social worker aids DeCola in forging meaningful social and community ties, potentially guiding him towards community centers, interest-based groups, or volunteer opportunities, thereby nurturing a supportive network and enriching DeCola's social life.

As DeCola makes strides in his recovery, the social worker assists in assessing the effectiveness of implemented interventions and planning for forthcoming needs. This involves setting new objectives, gradually phasing out certain services, or shifting the focus to other life areas warranting attention.

This collaborative and adaptable engagement with a social worker is designed to empower DeCola, aiming to elevate his well-being to a point where he can lead a fulfilling life backed by the necessary tools and support network to sustain his mental health.

DeCola and His General Counsellor

DeCola's engagement with a general counselor marks another phase in his mental health recovery, characterized by a structured yet empathetic approach tailored to his unique situation. The journey begins with an initial consultation, where the counselor creates a welcoming environment for DeCola to articulate his concerns and set the stage for a trusting therapeutic alliance.

Following this, a comprehensive assessment delves into the intricacies of DeCola's experiences, emotional landscape, and the challenges he faces. This in-depth exploration aids in uncovering the roots of his concerns and his strengths, shaping the path forward.

Setting goals is a collaborative effort, with DeCola and the counselor defining clear, attainable objectives that resonate with DeCola's aspirations for therapy. Whether it's managing stress, enhancing emotional well-being, or improving personal relationships, these goals guide the therapeutic journey.

A tailored therapeutic plan emerges from this collaborative groundwork, detailing the strategies and corresponding interventions that are employed. This plan is dynamic, adapting to DeCola's evolving needs as therapy progresses.

DeCola then embarks on regular therapy sessions, a safe space where he and the counselor engage in meaningful dialogue, explore underlying thoughts and emotions, and employ therapeutic techniques designed to foster healing and growth.

The counselor introduces various therapeutic tools and exercises suited to DeCola's challenges, from cognitive-behavioral tactics to mindfulness practices. These interventions aim to help DeCola navigate his difficulties, transform unhelpful thought patterns, and cultivate new, constructive behaviors.

Reflective practice becomes a cornerstone of their sessions, encouraging DeCola to ponder his inner world and behavioral responses. This reflection deepens his self-awareness and promotes personal insight, key components of lasting change.

Periodic reviews of DeCola's progress allow both him and the counselor to acknowledge successes, confront persisting obstacles, and refine the therapeutic approach to ensure it remains aligned with his journey.

The counselor equips DeCola with a variety of coping strategies and life skills, empowering him to manage his mental health autonomously and resiliently face life's ups and downs.

As DeCola approaches his therapeutic goals, the counselor thoughtfully guides him toward the conclusion of their sessions, focusing on sustaining his achievements and preparing him for future challenges.

The therapy culminates in a final session that offers both reflection and closure, celebrating the strides DeCola has made and reinforcing his readiness to continue his journey with confidence and self-assurance. Throughout this process, the counsellor's unwavering support and guidance provide DeCola with a foundation of understanding, healing, and growth, pivotal to his journey towards mental wellness.

DeCola and His Occupational Therapist

DeCola's collaboration with an Occupational Therapist (which DeCola prefers to tag OT as it coincides with the initials of the therapist) becomes a cornerstone in his mental health recovery, particularly as he navigates the daily challenges posed by his condition. This therapeutic partnership kicks off with an in-depth evaluation where the OT assesses DeCola's functional capabilities, daily challenges, and personal aspirations, laying the groundwork for a customized recovery roadmap.

Together, they chart out DeCola's recovery goals, focusing on enhancing his daily functioning and enriching his engagement in meaningful activities. These goals span from refining day-to-day task management to bolstering his performance in professional or academic settings and fostering more dynamic social and leisure engagements.

With these goals as their guide, the OT crafts a bespoke intervention plan, pinpointing strategies and activities tailored to DeCola's specific needs. This plan aims to empower DeCola with essential life skills, adapt tasks to his capabilities, and, when necessary, introduce adaptive tools to ease his daily routines.

DeCola then embarks on a series of therapeutic activities, carefully selected to resonate with his interests and aimed at improving his functional skills. These activities not only enhance his competency and self-reliance but also instill a sense of achievement and bolster his self-esteem.

The OT ensures that DeCola's therapy resonates with his values and lifestyle, enhancing his motivation and engagement. This personalized approach ensures that DeCola finds genuine fulfillment in the therapeutic process.

Education plays a pivotal role in DeCola's journey, with the OT equipping him with strategies to manage his mental health symptoms effectively within the context of his daily activities. This education spans stress reduction techniques, mood management during tasks, and organizing his environment to support his mental well-being.

As DeCola advances, the OT progressively intensifies the complexity of the tasks, introducing new challenges to foster resilience and adaptability, ensuring a continuum of personal growth and development.

Regular reviews and adjustments to the therapy plan are integral, allowing DeCola and the OT to gauge progress and tweak the approach to align with DeCola's evolving needs and aspirations.

Approaching the culmination of his therapy, the OT assists DeCola in devising a transition plan, outlining strategies for maintaining his therapeutic gains, tapping into community resources for continued support, and preparing for potential future hurdles.

The therapy concludes when DeCola achieves his set goals and is determined to maximize the benefits of occupational therapy. The OT offers follow-up sessions to ensure DeCola's sustained progress post-therapy.

Engaging with an OT equips DeCola with the skills and strategies to tackle the practicalities of living with a mental health condition, emphasizing his participation in daily tasks and pursuits that imbue his life with purpose and joy. This collaborative and personalized therapeutic journey fosters a holistic approach to DeCola's mental health recovery, centered around his unique needs, strengths, and aspirations.

DeCola and His Peer Support Therapist

DeCola's mental health recovery journey is significantly enriched through his engagement with a Peer Support Specialist, an individual who brings personal experience of overcoming mental health challenges to the table, coupled with specialized training to guide others through similar journeys. Their collaboration unfolds through a series of meaningful interactions:

The partnership ignites with DeCola's introduction to the Peer Support Specialist, setting the stage for a relationship grounded in trust and mutual respect. This initial meeting is pivotal in laying the foundation for open and empathetic communication.

In a gesture of solidarity and understanding, the Peer Support Specialist shares their mental health journey, offering DeCola a mirror to his own experiences and reinforcing that he is not alone in his struggles. This shared narrative fosters a deep sense of connection and relatability.

Together, they embark on a goal-setting expedition, pinpointing DeCola's aspirations and milestones he wishes to achieve throughout his recovery. These objectives span a spectrum of personal, social, and professional domains tailored to DeCola's unique life context.

The essence of their relationship is collaborative with mutual openness, with the Peer Support Specialist serving as an example of empathy, encouragement, and validation. This dynamic ensures DeCola feels genuinely supported and valued in expressing himself fully.

DeCola is introduced to a variety of coping mechanisms and resilience-building tools that have proven effective in the Peer Support Specialist's journey and within the broader recovery community. These strategies encompass stress management, interpersonal communication, team building and practical problem-solving skills.

Navigating the complex landscape of mental health services and resources becomes less daunting with the Peer Support Specialist by DeCola's side, guiding him to additional support systems that can amplify his recovery process.

A critical aspect of their collaboration is empowering DeCola to advocate for his needs and preferences, ensuring he feels confident and prepared to communicate effectively with healthcare providers and within other spheres of his life.

Peer support groups play a vital role in DeCola's journey, offering a platform for shared experiences, mutual support, and a sense of belonging. Facilitated or recommended by the Peer Support Specialist, these groups help dissolve feelings of isolation and provide collective wisdom on navigating mental health challenges.

Regular check-ins allow for reflection on DeCola's progress, acknowledging achievements and addressing emerging hurdles. This consistent support helps sustain DeCola's momentum and motivation on the path to recovery.

As DeCola evolves and his needs shift, the Peer Support Specialist adapts the support offered, ensuring it remains aligned with DeCola's current state and future aspirations. This flexibility is key to providing relevant and impactful guidance.

Ultimately, the Peer Support Specialist aims to equip DeCola with the confidence, skills, and knowledge to independently manage his mental health and continue progressing toward his recovery goals.

As DeCola moves forward, they collaboratively devise a forward-looking plan, setting new goals and strategies to maintain and build upon the mental health gains achieved.

In this unique therapeutic relationship, DeCola finds not just support, but a reflection of his potential for growth and recovery, instilling hope and driving him to embrace his journey with renewed vigor and self-assurance.

DeCola and His Art Counsellor

Embarking on a journey to navigate the complexities of addiction and concurrent mental health challenges, DeCola finds a guiding light in the form of an art counselor. This unique therapeutic alliance commences with a thorough assessment, where the counselor gauges the depth of DeCola's addiction and its interplay with his psychological well-being, setting the stage for a tailored recovery path.

The initial phase of therapy is dedicated to fostering a bond of trust and understanding, establishing a foundational rapport that encourages open communication and vulnerability. This relationship is instrumental for DeCola, providing him with a secure platform to express his struggles and aspirations.

Jointly, DeCola and his counselor articulate clear, realistic goals that pave the way for his recovery. These objectives are custom fit to DeCola's journey, encompassing composure, mental health enhancement, relational healing, and an overall uplift in life quality.

With these goals as their north star, a comprehensive treatment plan comes to life, weaving together individualized counseling, therapeutic group interactions, and engagement with supportive communities. This multifaceted strategy is designed to address the roots of DeCola's addiction and foster resilience against relapse.

Central to their sessions is the exploration of underlying emotional and psychological terrains that may be fueling DeCola's addiction. Through art therapy, DeCola delves into past traumas, current stressors, and emotional battles, finding expression and understanding in the creative process.

Equipped with new coping mechanisms and resilience strategies, DeCola learns to navigate life's stresses and triggers without falling back on substance use. These tools range from mindfulness and stress management to effective communication and problem-solving skills, all tailored to support his unique recovery journey.

A cornerstone of their work together is crafting a robust relapse prevention blueprint. This involves identifying potential relapse triggers, strategizing around them, and laying out a clear action plan should challenges arise, ensuring DeCola remains steadfast in his recovery path.

The counselor's role extends to bolstering DeCola's motivation and commitment to change, employing techniques like motivational interviewing to keep DeCola focused on the benefits of self-control and aligned with his core values and aspirations.

An integral part of DeCola's healing journey is building a network of support, encompassing family, friends, recovery peers, and community resources. This network not only offers emotional backing but also enriches DeCola's sense of belonging and social connectivity.

As DeCola progresses, his journey is punctuated by regular reviews and adaptations of his treatment plan, ensuring that his recovery evolves in harmony with his changing needs and circumstances.

Gradually, as DeCola nears his recovery milestones, the counselor prepares him for the transition from intensive therapy to a more self-directed phase of maintenance and growth, focusing on the sustainability of his recovery gains.

Post-therapy, follow-up sessions or check-ins are arranged to provide DeCola with ongoing support, helping him navigate any new challenges and reinforcing his commitment to a life of recovery and well-being.

Through the innovative and empathetic approach of art therapy, DeCola's journey with his counselor becomes a transformative and colorful venture, intertwining creativity with recovery to chart a course toward healing and self-discovery.

DeCola and His Music Counsellor

DeCola's recovery journey is enriched by the inclusion of music therapy, offering him a harmonious blend of self-expression, emotional exploration, and therapeutic growth. The collaboration with a music counselor unfolds through a series of carefully orchestrated steps, each resonating with DeCola's affinity for poems expressed via rhythm, rhymes and pace.

The journey commences with an initial consultation, where the music counselor delves into DeCola's musical inclinations, his mental health landscape, and the potential of music therapy to harmonize his path to recovery. This foundational session aims to align the therapy with DeCola's unique needs and aspirations.

Goals are then set in harmony, with DeCola and the counselor composing objectives that strike a chord with his desired outcomes. Whether it's channeling emotions through music, lifting his spirits, or amplifying his self-esteem, these goals set the tone for the therapeutic process.

DeCola is then invited to engage with music in a way that feels most natural to him. Whether through listening, playing, composing, or improvising, the therapy is attuned to his comfort and connection with music, requiring no prior musical expertise but rather an openness to explore its therapeutic potential.

Within this melodic space, DeCola discovers avenues to voice his emotions and navigate his inner narratives, guided by the rhythms and melodies that emerge. This musical expression becomes a conduit for uncovering deeper emotional insights and fostering a profound understanding of his emotional self.

Post-session reflections with the counselor allow De-Cola to articulate his experiences, emotions, and the revelations stirred by the music. These discussions help tether his musical explorations to his broader mental health journey, weaving insights into the fabric of his recovery.

The counselor also introduces DeCola to music-centered including voice training exercises aimed at developing specific life skills. From relaxation techniques to enhancing focus or social interactions, these musical interventions are tailored to support DeCola's therapeutic goals and everyday resilience.

As DeCola progresses through his sessions, the therapeutic duet with his counselor regularly reviews and fine-tunes their approach, ensuring the therapy remains in harmony with his evolving needs and continues to be a source of strength and solace.

Realizing DeCola's poetic potential, the counselor gently prepares DeCola to embrace music as a sustaining force in his life beyond therapy, encouraging him to integrate musical practices into his self-care repertoire.

DeCola shared that his journey with the music therapist has been a deeply transformative experience, likening it to composing a symphony where each session added a new dimension to his understanding of music and himself. He emphasized that the journey was about discovering the essence of music's meaning to him, going beyond mere notes on a page.

DeCola recounted how they explored his musical passions, identifying the genres and instruments that resonated most with his soul. This process of exploration felt like piecing together a puzzle, revealing new aspects of himself with each discovery. DeCola appreciated the therapist's ability to tailor sessions to his tastes, making every moment profoundly impactful.

Skill development was highlighted as a cornerstone of their work together. DeCola was consequently empowered to venture into music compositions, and he credited his growing confidence to the therapist's support and celebration of each milestone, no matter how small.

DeCola was introduced to the wide array of roles within the music industry, expanding his vision for potential career paths in music beyond performing. This broadened his horizons and sparked curiosity about new opportunities.

Gaining real-world experience through internships, shadowing professionals, and participating in workshops became a pivotal part of DeCola's journey. He valued these opportunities for the invaluable insights and networking they provided.

Establishing an online presence was also a key focus, with the therapist guiding DeCola in crafting a personal brand that reflected his artistic identity. Each step forward in building his digital footprint was celebrated, marking his growing presence in the music community.

DeCola spoke about the exhilaration of performing, whether on local stages or online platforms and how these opportunities to connect with an audience became significant milestones in his journey.

Lastly, DeCola emphasized the importance of building connections within the music community. He learned the value of networking, finding mentors, and engaging with peers, which enriched his journey and underscored the idea that music is fundamentally about connection and shared experiences.

Reflecting on his experience, DeCola expressed profound gratitude for the journey with his therapist, describing
it as a voyage of self-discovery and growth, with music serving as a guiding compass in navigating his future.

In the harmonious sanctuary of music therapy, DeCola's
soul found its voice anew, transforming his path to recovery
into a melodic journey of self-discovery and healing. Guided
by the gentle expertise of his music counselor, each session
became a medium for DeCola to express his tumultuous
emotions and experiences through the universal language of
music, crafting a symphony that resonated with the depth of
his journey.

As the notes of his therapy wove through the tapestry of
his recovery, the embers of DeCola's passion for music were
gently fanned into a vibrant flame. The sessions, a blend of
melody and empathy, reawakened his innate musical gift,
guiding him to see music not just as a hobby but as a cardinal
focus for his future.

Amid this musical awakening, DeCola composed a
piece that stood as a testament to his journey—a personalized anthem that captured the essence of his resilience and
growth. This composition, born from the crucible of his

struggles and triumphs, was more than just a melody; it was a declaration of his triumph over adversity, a harmonic narrative of his ascent from the depths of despair to the heights of hope.

As the final chords of his music therapy sessions echoed into silence, DeCola stood at the threshold of a new beginning, his heart alight with the renewed love for music. This rekindled passion, coupled with the insights gleaned from his therapeutic journey, crystallized into a clear vision for his future—one where music was not only his solace but also his calling. In this symphony of healing and discovery, DeCola found not just the melody of his soul but the harmony of a purpose that promised to guide him through the rest of his life's composition. Hence, DeCola's anthem, a piece he proudly holds as his creation, emerged at the session's finale, eagerly awaiting its debut performance:

Verse 1:

In the quiet of the dawn, DeCola has found his song,

In the travail of the shadows, he danced towards the light,

He dares to take a stand, with every step of care,

With every stroke of caution, he paints his life in green.

Verse 2:

A melody of healing, in which all the notes belong.

With the rule of give and take, he finds himself a whole.

In the rhythm of the chorus, his strength renewed again,

Soprano blends with bass, and alto aligns with tenor.

Verse 3:

From the whispers in the darkness, the echoes reflect the
tune

His anthem sounds victorious in the day and through the
night.

With resilience as refrain, his mind begins to glow,

DeCola's triumphant anthem a true and peaceful rhyme.

Chorus:

Sing on, DeCola, your spirit's soaring high,

With every note and beat, your inner being awakes.

Your anthem rings with hope, its melody soft and sweet,

In the music of recovery, the lasting hope you find.

Chapter 7: Rediscovering Self-Care

DeCola's story highlights the critical realization that self-care extends beyond generic solutions, evolving into a tailored mosaic of practices that cater to the physical, mental, and spiritual aspects of one's being. This journey underscores the importance of patience, empathy towards oneself, and the bravery required to heed one's inner voice, thereby emphasizing that self-care is fundamentally an act of self-awareness and rebellion against life's inherent chaos.

The chapter sheds light on the transformative power of self-care, not as a luxury but as an essential strategy for fostering resilience and vitality. It points out that the effectiveness of any mental health recovery plan greatly depends on incorporating self-care as a core component. DeCola's engagement in proactive and well-integrated self-care routines not only complements the support received from professional and informal networks but also empowers him to take an active role in his healing process.

By interweaving self-care into his daily regimen, De-Cola constructs a solid personal support system that enhances the interventions undertaken for his mental health. This holistic approach amplifies the impact of self-care on the overall success of mental health recovery strategies, highlighting how such practices can offer individuals a renewed sense of control and zest for life.

In essence, DeCola's journey serves as a testament to the profound influence of individualized self-care in achieving mental well-being, presenting a reflective mirror for readers in their quest for self-nurturance and a balanced life amidst the tumult of existence.

DeCola's journey to manage his mental health extends beyond professional support, incorporating various self-care practices that play a vital role in his overall well-being. Some of the strategies he applied include:

DeCola's Mindfulness and Meditation

DeCola's self-care journey is profoundly anchored in the practice of mindfulness, a cornerstone that has brought significant transformation to his life. Central to this transformation is his daily dedication to mindfulness exercises, where he immerses himself in the present moment, setting aside time each day to engage in practices that ground him in the here and now.

His routine begins in a carefully curated space within his home, a tranquil haven designed for reflection and intro-spection. This space, equipped with a comfortable mat, sub-dued lighting, and the calming presence of greenery, serves as the backdrop for his morning rituals of mindfulness and meditation. Here, DeCola engages in breath-focused exer-cises, a foundational practice that steadies his mind and fos-ters a deep-seated sense of calm.

Transitioning from breathwork to meditation, DeCola explores a variety of techniques. He alternates between guided sessions that nurture narratives of self-kindness and silent meditations, where he observes his thoughts with a de-tached curiosity. This eclectic approach ensures his practice remains vibrant and responsive to his evolving needs.

Beyond the confines of his meditation nook, mindful-ness permeates DeCola's daily activities. Simple acts, like enjoying a cup of tea or strolling through a park, become op-portunities for mindful presence, allowing him to savor life's simple pleasures fully.

This consistent engagement with mindfulness has equipped DeCola with a robust resilience against stress and anxiety. Challenges that once seemed impossible now appear manageable, with the tumults of life met with a serene and steady response. This shift has not only facilitated his recovery but has also brought a newfound joy and serenity, enriching his life and relationships.

DeCola's engagement in meditation led him to a profound revelation, highlighting the vital role that mindfulness and inner peace play in our lives. This epiphany was intertwined with cherished memories of his late grandfather, a figure of immense love and wisdom in his life. He reflected on the depth of their bond, marked by a warmth and familiarity that only deep, unconditional love can foster. His grandfather was a man of devout faith who dedicated his life to the study, memorization, and application of Biblical teachings, embodying the principles he held dear.

DeCola's story underscores the transformative potential of mindfulness and meditation. By prioritizing these practices, he has navigated his recovery with grace, uncovering a deep sense of peace and fulfillment that extends beyond personal healing to enhance every aspect of his life.

This spiritual discipline, DeCola realized, was the cornerstone of his grandfather's unparalleled joy, contentment, and fulfillment. It became evident that these qualities were not merely coincidental but were the direct result of a life lived in alignment with profound spiritual truths and a deep commitment to inner tranquillity. His grandfather's serene demeanour, even in the face of death, spoke volumes about the tranquillity that guided his life. The peaceful smile he wore in his final moments was a testament to a life well-lived, filled with purpose and inner peace, offering a poignant reminder of the transformative power of meditation and mindfulness. DeCola's reflection on these aspects brought to light the essence of true fulfillment, both in life and at his death, underscoring the importance of cultivating a mindful and meditative practice.

DeCola's Physical Exercise

Physical wellness has emerged as a foundational element in DeCola's self-care regimen, reflecting a deep understanding of the symbiotic relationship between physical activity and mental well-being. He has wholeheartedly embraced exercise as a pivotal component of his recovery, finding in it a powerful means to bolster his physical strength, mitigate stress, and enhance his mood. Every walk in the park and each workout session is more than mere physical exertion; it's a deliberate act of self-care and a testament to his dedication to holistic health.

DeCola's journey, however, is marked by its fair share of challenges and learning curves. The quest to discover activities that truly nourish his spirit involves navigating through moments of doubt and adjusting to changes in his preferences and needs. What once brought joy might now feel like a chore, underscoring the evolving nature of self-care and the importance of adaptability and persistence.

Exercise, in particular, has evolved from a reluctant obligation to an integral and cherished part of his daily routine. The rhythmic patterns of physical activity, whether through the steady cadence of running or the fluid movements of yoga, have become powerful expressions of resilience and an affirmation of the inner strength that DeCola possesses.

His approach to exercise is characterized by variety and balance, ensuring a holistic impact on his well-being. Mornings might find him jogging through the tranquility of the local park, embracing the solitude and the refreshing embrace of the dawn air. These runs are not just physical endeavors but reflective journeys that parallel the path of his personal growth and healing.

Strength training also plays a significant role in DeCola's fitness regimen, offering him a structured outlet to challenge and fortify his physical capabilities. The systematic nature of weightlifting becomes a metaphor for overcoming life's obstacles, with each repetition reinforcing his resilience and capacity for endurance.

Yoga, with its emphasis on mindfulness and the harmony between body and breath, offers DeCola a peaceful retreat from the world's hustle. It's within the stillness of his yoga practice that he finds a profound sense of inner peace and balance, further illustrating the multifaceted benefits of his physical activities.

Beyond the personal gains, DeCola's commitment to fitness has ripple effects, inspiring his community to recognize the value of incorporating movement into their lives. His journey underscores the transformative potential of regular physical exercise, not only for enhancing physical health but also for its invaluable contributions to mental and emotional wellness.

In sum, DeCola's holistic engagement with physical exercise underscores its vital role in nurturing the body, mind, and spirit. His story is a compelling testament to the power of a well-rounded fitness routine in forging a path toward a more balanced, fulfilling, and resilient life.

DeCola found a unique synergy in combining his physical exercises with the vibrant accompaniment of percussive music, rhythm, and rhymes, which not only invigorated his workouts but also sparked his creative energy. This harmonious blend of movement and music became a fertile ground for his artistic expression, allowing him to delve deeper into his poetic and musical compositions. The rhythmic beats and melodies provided a backdrop that inspired him, synchronizing with his movements to enhance his focus and creativity.

This innovative approach to exercise transformed his sessions into a dynamic and immersive experience, where every movement was infused with a sense of purpose and artistic exploration. The physical exertion, paired with the stimulating sounds, acted as a catalyst for his creative processes, enabling him to channel his thoughts and emotions into written and musical forms more fluidly and expressively.

As a result, DeCola not only reaped the physical benefits of consistent and engaging workouts but also experienced a profound enrichment of his artistic abilities. This unique integration of physical and creative endeavors underscored the multifaceted benefits of a well-rounded approach to personal development, where the body and the mind are harmoniously engaged in pursuits that nourish and elevate one's overall well-being.

DeCola's Healthy Eating Habits

Nutrition has emerged as a key component of DeCola's self-care regime, fundamentally shaping his journey toward holistic wellness. Recognizing the profound connection between what he consumes and his mental and physical state, DeCola has embraced a dietary approach that is as nurturing as it is healing. Guided by insights from healthcare professionals, he now views his meals as vital sources of nourishment, each selection contributing significantly to his well-being.

Embracing the principle that food serves as his body's medicine, DeCola's diet is rich in whole, unprocessed foods, a colorful array of fruits, vegetables, lean proteins, and whole grains. This diverse palette not only feeds his body with essential nutrients but also brings joy and creativity into his daily routine. Cooking has transformed into a therapeutic activity for DeCola, a mindful practice where the preparation of each meal is an act of self-care.

At the heart of DeCola's nutritional philosophy lies the application of his essential body's needs. He practices intuitive eating, honoring his hunger signals and respecting his fullness, which fosters a peaceful and fulfilling relationship with food. This approach steers clear of restrictive dieting, advocating instead for a sustainable and enjoyable eating experience.

DeCola also values diversity in his diet, understanding that a variety of foods ensures a comprehensive intake of nutrients essential for cognitive function and emotional equilibrium. He regularly explores different cuisines and ingredients, making each meal an opportunity for discovery and delight while ensuring his body and mind are well-supported.

Hydration is another pillar of DeCola's nutritional strategy. Consistent water intake is crucial for him, aiding in focus and mood stabilization. He makes a conscious effort to stay hydrated, recognizing its role in supporting his overall health.

The transformative impact of these dietary changes on DeCola's life is unmistakable. Improved physical energy has invigorated his participation in daily activities and exercise, while the stabilizing effects on his mood have ushered in a more consistent and positive emotional state. Through mindful nutrition, DeCola has found a key ingredient in his recipe for a balanced and vibrant life.

Determined to achieve the pinnacle of health and wellness, DeCola engaged in a thorough consultation with his General Practitioner (GP), keen on unravelling the intricate tapestry of his body's unique needs. This deep dive into his physiological blueprint was not merely routine; it was a quest for a nutrition strategy tailored just for him, transcending the generic dietary guidelines that often fall short of individual complexities.

With meticulous care, his GP conducted a holistic evaluation, weaving together DeCola's medical narratives, current health dynamics, and even the subtle whispers of his genetic heritage. This rich tapestry of information became the cornerstone for devising a nutritional plan as unique as De-Cola himself. It wasn't just about eating healthily; it was about eating intelligently, in harmony with his body's specific requirements and current medical treatments.

Heeding the insights derived from this comprehensive assessment, DeCola embarked on a culinary journey tailored to fortify his health. The revelation of his propensity for low iron levels led to a deliberate inclusion of iron-packed wonders like leafy greens, hearty legumes, and lean proteins, each bite augmented by the vitamin C burst from citrus fruits to ensure maximum iron absorption. Meanwhile, the blueprint for heart health was etched with omega-3-rich selections like succulent salmon and crunchy walnuts, complemented by a vibrant array of fruits, vegetables, and grains, each component meticulously chosen to support a robust heart.

However, DeCola's personalized menu went beyond mere nutrient optimization. With his GP's guidance, it was finely tuned to merge seamlessly with his current medications, sidestepping potential food-drug interactions that could compromise their efficacy or provoke unwelcome side effects. For instance, if grapefruit could interfere with his medication, it was prudently replaced with alternatives that offered similar nutritional benefits without the risk.

This enlightened approach to nutrition, grounded in personalization and medical insight, transformed DeCola's diet into a powerful ally in his wellness journey. It was not just about avoiding the adverse effects of a one-size-fits-all diet; it was about embracing a way of eating that resonated with his body's unique rhythm, enhancing his vitality, mental acuity, and overall well-being. In this harmonious blend of science and personalization, DeCola found not just a diet but a lifestyle that echoed his body's deepest needs and aspirations for health.

DeCola's Adequate Sleep

Recognizing the significance of maintaining healthy boundaries became a crucial aspect of DeCola's self-care journey. He learned the value of saying no to obligations that could deplete his resources, treating his time and energy as sacred. This understanding allowed him to cultivate a life where relaxation is not a mere indulgence but a vital element of his well-being.

Central to his wellness strategy is the role of sleep, regarded by DeCola as essential to his health. He acknowledges the deep influence of restful sleep on his mental sharpness, emotional stability, and physical energy. To honor this, he has established a bedtime ritual that treats sleep with the reverence it deserves, ensuring his nights are conducive to healing and restoration.

DeCola adheres to a consistent sleep schedule, setting fixed times for going to bed and waking up. This routine has synchronized his internal clock, improving his ability to fall asleep and enhancing the quality of his rest. His evenings are characterized by a series of rituals aimed at preparing his mind and body for sleep, including dimming the lights to create a calming atmosphere and disconnecting from electronic devices to ease the transition from wakefulness to rest.

His bedroom is a sanctuary designed for tranquility, where pre-sleep routines such as a warm shower and the occasional herbal tea play a supportive role in signaling his body that it's time to wind down. Mindfulness and meditation are also integral to his nightly routine, aiding in the release of daily stresses and fostering a peaceful state of mind conducive to quality sleep.

The disciplined approach DeCola takes toward ensuring sufficient rest has yielded significant benefits. Mornings find him rejuvenated, with clarity of mind and a readiness to face the day's challenges with enthusiasm and a positive perspective. The consistency in his sleep pattern has not only bolstered his physical health but also enhanced his mental and emotional resilience, reducing instances of mood swings and cognitive fog.

Furthermore, DeCola's commitment to prioritizing sleep has served as an inspirational model to his community, highlighting the indispensable link between rest and overall health. His practices advocate for a cultural shift that reeval-

251

uates the importance of sleep, demonstrating its transformative effects on mental clarity, emotional balance, and vitality.

In summary, DeCola's profound respect for sleep as a
cornerstone of self-care underscores its critical impact on our
holistic health. His experiences illuminate the essential nature of rest in fostering a balanced and fulfilling life, where
sleep is treasured as a fundamental pillar of health and happiness.

DeCola's Journaling

Journaling has become an integral part of DeCola's self-
care routine, acting as both a reflective mirror and a guiding
map that captures the essence of his inner experiences and
life's journey. This practice transcends the act of simple rec-
ord-keeping; for DeCola, it is a sacred communion with his
innermost self, a cherished ritual that provides solace from
the daily grind.

In the tranquil moments of the evening, DeCola retreats
to a specially curated nook in his home, designed to foster
introspection with its comfortable ambiance and soothing
lighting. It is here, in this personal haven, that he engages

with his journal, a faithful repository of his thoughts, aspirations, and reflections.

The process of journaling for DeCola is one of unfiltered expression, where he allows his consciousness to spill onto the pages without restraint or judgment. This practice serves as a therapeutic release, enabling him to navigate the complex tapestry of emotions and experiences that define his day-to-day life. Often, it is through this candid outpouring that DeCola stumbles upon insights and revelations, uncovering truths hidden beneath the surface of his conscious mind.

Journaling also offers DeCola a platform for reflection, allowing him to revisit past entries, acknowledge his growth, and identify areas in need of attention. This introspective dialogue with himself is invaluable, fostering a sense of gratitude and understanding of the journey he has undertaken.

Furthermore, DeCola's journal is a tool for intention setting and progress tracking, each entry serving as a commitment to his goals and aspirations. This proactive aspect of journaling empowers him, turning his journal into a testament to his personal growth, adorned with markers of resilience and achievements.

The impact of journaling on DeCola's mental and emotional health is profound. It has become a cornerstone for stress relief and self-awareness, offering a sanctuary where he can lighten his emotional load and gain clarity. Through this practice, DeCola has cultivated a deeper sense of peace and understanding, equipping him to face life's challenges with grace and insight.

DeCola's dedication to journaling underscores the profound benefits of this practice, highlighting its capacity to offer clarity, strength, and a deeper connection to oneself. His journey through journaling serves as an inspiration, encouraging others to embark on their explorations of self through the written word, unlocking the potential for self-discovery and emotional resilience.

DeCola's Hobbies and Interests

Engaging in activities that he enjoys and that give him a sense of accomplishment, such as art, music, or gardening, provides DeCola with positive distractions and outlets for self-expression.

DeCola has discovered the transformative power of engaging with hobbies and interests, reigniting passions that mental health challenges had once dimmed. Activities like

254

painting, reading, and gardening have become more than leisure pursuits; they are lifelines to joy and a sense of purpose, affirming the richness of life beyond the shadows of mental illness.

In addition, DeCola has learned the crucial art of setting healthy boundaries, ensuring he doesn't overcommit and thus safeguarding his time and energy as invaluable assets. This discipline has enabled him to foster a lifestyle where relaxation and rejuvenation are not optional but essential pillars of his self-care routine.

A significant aspect of DeCola's journey involves delving into creative expressions such as poetry and music, which have become vital avenues for him to articulate and process his emotions. Through the nuanced language of poetry, he captures and communicates experiences and feelings that are otherwise elusive, finding solace and understanding in the rhythm and resonance of words.

Music, too, holds a special place in DeCola's heart, serving as both a source of comfort and a medium of expression. Whether strumming a guitar, immersing in favorite melodies, or crafting his compositions, music allows DeCola to connect with a universal language that transcends words yet speaks profoundly to human experience.

Interestingly, DeCola often blends his poetic endeavors with musical creativity, setting his verses to tunes. This synthesis of lyrics and rhymes not only enriches his artistic expression but also fosters a deeper connection with listeners, offering them a glimpse into his inner world.

These artistic pursuits provide DeCola not only with intrinsic satisfaction and personal growth but also with a sense of achievement and community connection, especially when sharing his work. The act of creation and the feedback he receives become sources of validation and shared human experience.

Moreover, DeCola finds poetry and music a constructive diversion from everyday stressors, a therapeutic outlet that renews his spirit and offers fresh perspectives on life's challenges.

Through his dedication to these hobbies, DeCola underscores the importance of engaging with one's passions as a way to enhance life's tapestry. His story exemplifies how creative pursuits can be a wellspring of joy, self-discovery, and resilience, enriching one's existence with meaning and fulfillment.

DeCola's Social Connections

As DeCola progresses through healing, fostering social connections transcends mere social activity; it's an essential lifeline that provides joy, understanding, and support, significantly enhancing his life. He places immense value on cultivating and rebuilding deep, meaningful relationships with both friends and family, recognizing these connections as foundational to his emotional health and resilience.

In today's rapid pace of life, DeCola is mindful not to let valuable relationships wane or to replace meaningful interactions with superficial digital communication. He actively seeks out genuine connections, ensuring that his interactions with loved ones are intentional and heartfelt.

DeCola's circle of friends is more than just a social network; it's a support system of individuals who share a deep mutual understanding and respect. These friends have been his pillars through various life challenges, celebrating his successes and providing comfort during difficult times. DeCola dedicates regular time to these pivotal relationships, connecting through phone calls, letters, or personal gatherings, valuing the quality of these interactions.

Family is particularly dear to DeCola, serving as a source of unwavering support and comfort. He ensures that family connections remain strong through frequent gatherings and communication, maintaining a close-knit bond even when separated by distance. Technology plays a crucial role in keeping these familial ties vibrant, allowing for a continuous share of life's significant and everyday moments.

Beyond his immediate social circle, DeCola extends his engagement to the broader community, participating in volunteer efforts and group activities that resonate with his interests. These broader interactions enrich his life with varied perspectives and contribute to a diverse and supportive community network.

The profound influence of these nurtured relationships on DeCola's well-being cannot be overstated. They afford him a sense of belonging and mutual understanding, serving as a beacon during times of solitude or uncertainty and reinforcing his sense of self-worth.

Additionally, these relationships act as reflective surfaces, revealing to DeCola his inherent qualities of love, resilience, and strength, especially in moments when he might doubt himself. They encourage his personal growth and provide a safety net in challenging times.

DeCola's intentional approach to maintaining social connections underscores the vital human need for community and mutual support. His life exemplifies the significant role that relationships play in achieving emotional fulfillment and leading a rich, meaningful life. Through his actions, DeCola highlights the enduring power and necessity of forging and nurturing bonds with others, illustrating the integral impact of social connections on our life's journey.

DeCola's Digital Detox

DeCola embraces a comprehensive view of well-being that meticulously incorporates detoxification as a pivotal component, transcending mere physical health also to address the digital dimensions of his existence. He firmly understands that in the contemporary landscape, health is a multifaceted concept where an array of environmental and digital pollutants can adversely affect one's wellness.

With a discerning eye toward the dual nature of digital connectivity, DeCola is committed to regular digital detox practices. He is fully conscious of the fact that, although digital platforms can foster connections, they also have the potential to encroach upon personal tranquillity and space. In response, he establishes clear boundaries for digital engagement, such as disabling notifications, allocating time to put away digital devices, or embracing entire days without screens, all in a bid to reclaim his focus and peace from the pervasive influence of digital life.

The impact of these digital detox practices on his well-being is profound, markedly reducing stress levels and enhancing the quality of his life. Through intentional digital breaks, DeCola cultivates moments of solitude and introspection, paving the way for creativity, deep-focused work, and mental clarity amid the constant digital chatter.

On the physical detox front, DeCola adopts a holistic strategy aimed at bolstering his body's natural detoxification processes. This involved integrating only safe detoxification practices, always under expert advice. His preference leans towards gentle, sustainable methods that enhance the body's innate detox pathways, thus invigorating his energy and resilience.

This deliberate detoxification approach mirrors De-Cola's broader philosophy on health and wellness, which acknowledges the intricate interplay between our physical, digital, and emotional spheres. By periodically disconnecting from the digital realm and aiding his body in its natural purification efforts, he not only diminishes stress but also enhances his connection with the immediate, tangible world more mindfully and healthfully.

DeCola's methodology highlights the essential practice of continually reassessing and recalibrating our engagement with both the tangible and virtual environments we navigate. His example serves as a compelling reminder of the necessity to balance our digital connectivity with strategic disengagement and to regard detoxification as an integral component of rejuvenation and an enriched life experience.

DeCola's Interest in Nature

DeCola cherishes nature not just as a venue for recreation but as an essential wellspring of well-being, a serene haven where he re-establishes his connection with the earth and, consequently, with his inner self. His profound appreciation for the natural world compels him to integrate nature into his daily routine, acknowledging its capacity to soothe the mind, elevate the soul, and energize the body.

DeCola's engagements with nature are deliberate and varied, ranging from tranquil walks in lush parks to challenging hikes and peaceful moments beside meandering streams. These interactions serve as a counterbalance to the hustle of daily life, providing him with a solid foundation in the here and now and a respite from life's pressures and distractions.

The tranquillity that nature bestows upon DeCola is unmistakable. Immersed in the gentle rustlings, the calm breezes, and nature's intricate wonders, he experiences a significant slowdown in his thoughts and a welcome relief from stress, enveloped in a serene calm that rejuvenates his spirit.

But the benefits DeCola derives from nature extend beyond mere peace; they encompass a deep-seated joy and vitality. The splendor of the natural landscape, from the vivid colors of flora to the expansive skies, ignites in him a sense of wonder and a profound appreciation for life's beauty, enriching his outdoor ventures with moments of awe and reverence.

These outdoor experiences also nurture DeCola's awareness of the intricate web of life, enhancing his sense of interconnectedness and responsibility towards the environment. This reflective understanding deepens the significance of his time in nature, imbuing it with a sense of purpose and belonging.

DeCola's commitment to immersing himself in nature underscores the restorative and transformative effects of the natural environment on our well-being. His practice highlights the importance of stepping out of our man-made surroundings to embrace the simplicity and grandeur of the natural world, offering a model for how such connections can foster healing, inspiration, and rejuvenation in our lives.

DeCola's Learning and Personal Development

DeCola embraces life as an ongoing odyssey of exploration and self-improvement, driven by a deep-seated commitment to continuous learning and personal growth. He views the acquisition of new knowledge and skills not just as hobbies but as integral components of his very essence, fueling a perpetual sense of intellectual curiosity and personal advancement that deeply enriches his existence.

His approach to learning is dynamic and broad, reflecting his conviction that growth can emerge from a wide array of experiences. Whether mastering the subtleties of a new language or demystifying the complexities of the latest technology, DeCola revels in the discovery process. Each new endeavor opens up vistas of understanding and possibility.

DeCola's dedication to self-improvement transcends cognitive pursuits, encompassing the realms of emotional and social competencies as well. He values emotional intelligence and interpersonal abilities as essential to both personal fulfillment and professional success, actively engaging in activities that challenge his viewpoints and foster introspection.

The rewards of DeCola's lifelong learning journey are multifaceted. Intellectually, he maintains a keen mental acuity and a diverse knowledge base that renders him an insightful and adaptable individual, attributes that confer a competitive edge in his professional life.

However, the true essence of DeCola's quest for self-development lies in the profound satisfaction and sense of competence it brings him. Each newly acquired skill or piece of knowledge represents a milestone on his path of self-discovery, weaving a rich mosaic of experiences that shape his identity and aspirations. This ongoing sense of achievement is a powerful motivator, propelling him forward in his quest for new learning opportunities.

Furthermore, DeCola's commitment to personal growth imparts resilience, enabling him to confront challenges with a blend of creativity and assurance born of his varied experiences and skills. This adaptability not only aids him in navigating life's vicissitudes but also stands as a beacon of inspiration for others, underscoring the value of lifelong learning.

In sum, DeCola's active engagement in continuous learning and self-development exemplifies the profound impact that a curious and open mindset can have on one's life. His journey underscores that personal growth extends beyond formal education, permeating every facet of life and offering endless opportunities for those who pursue it with zeal and determination. Through his example, DeCola highlights the pathway to a life enriched by unceasing discovery, skill acquisition, and, most importantly, an enduring sense of personal achievement.

By integrating these self-care practices into his daily life, DeCola takes proactive steps towards managing his mental health, complementing the support he receives from mental health professionals.

Chapter 8: Building Resilience

DeCola's mental health recovery journey showcases an intriguing paradox: embracing vulnerability becomes a profound source of resilience. This counterintuitive discovery—that openness to vulnerability can fortify inner strength—reshapes DeCola's approach to life's challenges and his understanding of personal growth.

By confronting and sharing his vulnerabilities, DeCola engages in authentic self-examination, fostering deep self-awareness. This self-awareness, the foundation of resilience, equips him with a clear understanding of his strengths and limitations, enabling him to navigate life with greater confidence and adaptability.

Sharing his vulnerabilities amplifies DeCola's resilience. Opening up about his struggles lightens his emotional burden and cultivates a supportive community. These connections reinforce that he is not alone, providing a network of support that bolsters his resilience. This communal strength empowers DeCola to face adversities with the knowledge that he has allies.

Moreover, DeCola's embrace of vulnerability challenges and reshapes his perception of strength. He learns that true resilience is not about maintaining an invulnerable façade but about the courage to be seen with all inherent imperfections. This redefinition of strength fosters a more sustainable form of resilience rooted in authenticity and acceptance of life's unpredictability.

Vulnerability also catalyzes personal growth, a key component of resilience. Each time DeCola confronts a challenge or shares his inner world, he expands his emotional and psychological boundaries. This continuous growth enhances his capacity to adapt to new situations, making him more resilient in the face of future challenges.

Additionally, DeCola's vulnerability-induced resilience increases his capacity for empathy, both towards himself and others. This empathy enriches his interactions and relationships, providing a foundation of mutual understanding and support. These strengthened relationships contribute to a support system that enhances his resilience.

In essence, DeCola's journey reveals the profound connection between vulnerability and resilience. Embracing vulnerability fosters deeper self-awareness, redefines strength, cultivates a supportive community, and encourages continuous growth. Through vulnerability, DeCola discovers a more authentic, empathetic, and adaptable form of resilience, equipping him with the inner resources needed to navigate the complexities of life and mental health recovery.

Central to this narrative is DeCola's exploration of lifestyle changes that underpin resilience. With newfound awareness from his therapeutic journey and self-care practices, DeCola integrates nurturing and sustainable habits into daily life. Nutrition gains new significance as he discovers its impact on mood and energy. Sleep, once undervalued, becomes a sacred ritual for healing and rejuvenation. DeCola learns to balance daily hustle with moments of rest and reflection, sustaining his mental and emotional well-being.

The narrative deepens as DeCola re-evaluates and strengthens his support systems. Recognizing the power of connection, he nurtures relationships that offer reciprocal understanding and support. Leaning into these bonds during moments of doubt, DeCola draws strength from shared experiences and collective wisdom. He also sets boundaries to protect his energy and well-being, fostering healthier and more meaningful connections.

Coping strategies become DeCola's arsenal against life's challenges. Through trial and reflection, he curates techniques ranging from deep breathing to cognitive reframing, transforming distortions into empowering affirmations. Journaling provides introspection, a space for DeCola to dialogue with himself, unravel fears, and celebrate victories.

A pivotal aspect of DeCola's journey is learning to anticipate and navigate potential triggers. Combining mindfulness and strategic planning, he recognizes stress and anxiety harbingers, proactively engaging coping strategies to soften their impact. This dance of anticipation and action empowers DeCola to remain steadfast in adversity.

"Building Resilience" is not just a chapter in DeCola's story; it is a testament to the human capacity for growth and adaptation. It showcases the intricate process of constructing a resilient self, fortified with the strength to face pain, learn from it, and emerge with deeper purpose and vitality. DeCola's journey reminds us that resilience is not innate but crafted through choices, efforts, and unwavering belief in our ability to endure and thrive.

Building upon these foundational practices, DeCola fortifies his resilience with a comprehensive and nuanced approach. This expanded framework sustains him through recovery and equips him to thrive amidst life's inevitable challenges.

DeCola's Emotional Regulation

DeCola's journey towards mental health recovery is significantly enhanced by his dedication to what he learned from his specialists coined emotional regulation". Recognizing the pivotal role emotions play in his well-being, DeCola commits to developing a nuanced understanding of his emotional landscape and the skills necessary to navigate it effectively. This commitment involves a proactive approach to learning and applying various techniques that help him maintain emotional equilibrium, even in the face of life's inevitable stressors.

One of the foundational techniques DeCola incorporates into his daily routine is deep breathing. By focusing on his breath, he creates a space of calm within himself, slowing down the whirlwind of thoughts and emotions that can often feel overwhelming. This practice of deep breathing becomes a quick-access tool for DeCola, offering him an immediate way to center himself whenever he senses the stirrings of emotional upheaval.

Progressive muscle relaxation is another strategy De-Cola finds particularly useful. Through this technique, he systematically works through different muscle groups in his body, tensing and then relaxing them. This not only helps in releasing the physical manifestation of stress but also serves as a metaphor for letting go of emotional tension. The physical act of relaxation cues his mind to follow suit, easing emotional stress and fostering a sense of bodily and mental harmony.

Positive visualization acts as a powerful ally in DeCola's emotional regulation toolkit. He often takes time to envision scenarios where he navigates challenging situations with calm and confidence. This practice of mental rehearsal strengthens his belief in his ability to manage difficult emotions and situations, effectively rewiring his responses to stress. By visualizing positive outcomes, DeCola nurtures a mindset that is more resilient and optimistic, further supporting his emotional stability.

These techniques, while diverse, share a common goal: they empower DeCola to take a step back from the immediacy of his emotions and assess them with clarity and composure. This ability to pause and reflect before reacting ensures that his responses to stressors are thoughtful and constructive rather than impulsive or destructive. The skills DeCola develops in emotional regulation not only serve him in moments of acute stress but also contribute to a more balanced and fulfilling life where emotions are experienced fully yet managed wisely.

DeCola's commitment to emotional regulation is a testament to his understanding that true resilience lies not in avoiding emotions but in navigating them with awareness and skill. By cultivating these capabilities, he ensures that his journey toward mental health recovery is marked by an increasing ability to face life's challenges with grace, strength, and emotional intelligence.

DeCola's Cognitive Reframing

DeCola's mental health recovery is significantly shaped by his engagement with what his psychologist referred to as "cognitive reframing", a powerful technique that allows him to alter his perspective on difficult situations. By consciously choosing to view challenges not as insurmountable obstacles but as opportunities for growth and learning, DeCola transforms the way he interacts with potential stressors, turning them into catalysts for personal development and resilience building.

This process of cognitive reframing involves DeCola stepping back from his initial, often automatic, reactions to stressful situations and examining them through a different lens. For instance, when faced with a setback, instead of succumbing to feelings of failure or disappointment, DeCola asks himself what he can learn from the experience. This deliberate shift in focus from the negative aspects to the potential positives changes the emotional impact of the situation. It not only diminishes the stress and anxiety that the challenge might have originally provoked but also empowers DeCola with a sense of control and agency over his response.

Moreover, by consistently practicing cognitive reframing, DeCola begins to internalize a growth-oriented mindset. This mindset champions the belief that every experience, especially the challenging ones, holds intrinsic value for learning and self-improvement. Such a perspective fosters resilience, as DeCola comes to understand that setbacks are not endpoints but rather integral parts of the journey toward growth. This realization imbues him with the strength to face future challenges with a more constructive and optimistic outlook.

Cognitive reframing also contributes to DeCola's emotional regulation, as it directly impacts how he emotionally processes events. By reinterpreting potentially negative situations as opportunities, the intensity of negative emotions associated with those situations diminishes, making them more manageable and less likely to trigger overwhelming stress or anxiety.

Furthermore, this technique enhances DeCola's problem-solving skills. Viewing challenges through the lens of growth and opportunity encourages a more creative and flexible approach to overcoming obstacles. This adaptability is a key component of resilience, enabling DeCola to navigate the complexities of life with greater ease and confidence.

In essence, cognitive reframing is a transformative tool in DeCola's mental health recovery arsenal. It allows him to reorient his perspective towards a more growth-focused and resilient outlook, turning potential stressors into valuable lessons. This shift not only mitigates the immediate impact of challenges but also contributes to a broader pattern of personal development, emotional regulation, and enhanced problem-solving abilities, all of which are foundational to his journey toward lasting well-being.

DeCola's Goal Setting and Achievement

DeCola's engagement with goal setting and achievement plays a crucial role in his mental health recovery journey. By identifying and working towards clear, attainable objectives, he crafts a structured path for his recovery and personal development. This approach not only provides direction but also instills a sense of purpose and motivation, driving him forward even in the face of challenges.

The act of setting goals allows DeCola to break down his broader recovery aspirations into manageable, concrete steps. Whether it's improving his emotional regulation, deepening his understanding of cognitive reframing, or enhancing his social connections, each goal serves as a milestone in his journey. This segmentation transforms the sometimes overwhelming task of recovery into a series of achievable targets, making the process more approachable and less daunting.

Achieving these goals, regardless of their scale, is pivotal in reinforcing DeCola's sense of self-efficacy. Every completed objective serves as tangible evidence of his ability to effect change in his life, bolstering his confidence in his capabilities. This sense of accomplishment is vital for DeCola's self-esteem, counteracting any feelings of helplessness or stagnation that might arise during the recovery process.

Moreover, the practice of setting and achieving goals contributes to DeCola's resilience. Each accomplished goal not only marks a step forward in his recovery but also strengthens his belief in his ability to overcome obstacles. This cycle of setting, pursuing, and achieving objectives builds a resilient mindset, equipping DeCola with the persistence and optimism needed to navigate future challenges.

Furthermore, the process of goal achievement is inherently linked to DeCola's growth and self-discovery. As he works towards his objectives, he inevitably encounters new experiences and insights that contribute to his personal development. This continuous learning and adaptation are key aspects of his recovery, fostering a dynamic and evolving sense of self.

Goal setting and achievement also provide DeCola with a mechanism for self-reflection and adjustment. By regularly reviewing his goals and the progress made towards them, he can assess what strategies are effective and where adjustments may be needed. This reflective practice ensures that his recovery journey remains aligned with his evolving needs and circumstances, allowing for flexibility and adaptability in his approach.

In essence, goal setting and achievement are integral to DeCola's mental health recovery. They offer a structured approach to his journey, imbuing it with direction, motivation, and a sense of purpose. The act of achieving these goals reinforces his self-efficacy and resilience while also facilitating continuous personal growth and adaptation. Through this process, DeCola navigates his recovery with a proactive and empowered stance, steadily building towards a future of well-being and fulfillment.

DeCola's Gratitude Practice

DeCola's incorporation of daily gratitude practice into his routine marks a significant stride in his mental health recovery. By taking time each day to reflect on and document the things he is thankful for, DeCola cultivates a habit that

gradually reorients his focus from the difficulties and challenges he faces to the positive aspects of his life. This seemingly simple practice has profound implications for his overall outlook and resilience.

This daily ritual of acknowledging gratitude allows De-
Cola to illuminate the often-overlooked positives that per-
meate his life. Whether it's appreciating the support of a
friend, the beauty of a quiet moment, or the progress he's
made in his recovery journey, each act of gratitude serves to
highlight the abundance of blessings surrounding him. This
shift in focus is not about denying or minimizing the challenges he faces but rather about balancing his perspective to
include the full spectrum of his experiences.

The consistent recognition of the positive aspects of his
life fosters a sense of abundance and well-being in DeCola.
Over time, this practice seeds a more optimistic outlook,
countering tendencies toward negativity and despair. The
positive emotions elicited by gratitude, such as joy, contentment, and appreciation, act as a counterbalance to the stress
and anxiety that can accompany mental health challenges,
providing a more stable emotional foundation.

Moreover, DeCola's gratitude practice contributes to his resilience by reinforcing a sense of connectedness and belonging. As he reflects on the people and experiences for which he is grateful, he strengthens his appreciation for the support network that surrounds him and recognizes his place within a larger community. This awareness of interconnection bolsters his resilience, reminding him that he is not alone in his journey and that there are many sources of support and joy in his life.

Furthermore, engaging in gratitude helps DeCola develop a greater appreciation for the progress he has made in his recovery. By acknowledging and celebrating the small victories and positive developments, he reinforces his sense of agency and accomplishment. This acknowledgment of progress, no matter how incremental, fuels his motivation to continue his path of healing and growth.

The practice of gratitude also has a grounding effect on DeCola, anchoring him in the present moment and encouraging a mindful approach to life. By focusing on the here and now, he reduces the tendency to dwell on past regrets or future anxieties, further contributing to his emotional stability and resilience.

In essence, DeCola's daily gratitude practice is a corner-stone of his mental health recovery, fostering a positive and balanced outlook that underpins his resilience. By regularly acknowledging and appreciating the blessings in his life, he cultivates a sense of well-being, connectedness, and appreciation for the journey, all of which are instrumental in building a robust foundation for his continued growth and healing.

DeCola's Willingness to Own Professional Support

DeCola's openness to seeking support from mental health professionals is a key component of his recovery journey. This willingness to engage with therapists or counselors, when necessary, provides him with a wealth of resources that significantly enhance his ability to navigate the complexities of mental health challenges. The professional guidance he receives acts as a catalyst for growth, offering him tools and insights that bolster his resilience.

Engaging with a mental health professional offers DeCola a structured environment where he can explore and understand his thoughts, emotions, and behaviors in depth. This exploration is guided by the expertise of the therapist, who brings a wealth of knowledge about mental health, offering strategies and therapeutic approaches tailored to DeCola's specific needs. This personalized guidance is invaluable, as it addresses the nuances of his experiences and provides targeted interventions that foster healing and growth.

The coping strategies DeCola learns through therapy or counseling are vital tools in his recovery arsenal. These strategies, ranging from cognitive-behavioral techniques to mindfulness practices, equip him with practical methods for managing stress, regulating emotions, and challenging negative thought patterns. By incorporating these strategies into his daily life, DeCola enhances his ability to navigate life's ups and downs with greater ease and stability.

Moreover, the external perspective offered by a mental health professional provides DeCola with invaluable insights that he might not have arrived at on his own. This fresh viewpoint can help him identify blind spots in his thinking or behavior, offering new ways of understanding and approaching his challenges. This external perspective often brings clarity and objectivity to situations that may feel overwhelming or confusing when navigated alone.

Therapy also provides DeCola with a safe and confidential space where he can express his thoughts and feelings openly, without fear of judgment. This aspect of therapy is crucial, as it allows him to explore and express vulnerabilities that may be difficult to share in other contexts. The therapeutic relationship itself, built on trust and empathy, becomes a source of support and validation, reinforcing DeCola's sense of being understood and accepted.

Additionally, the therapeutic process often involves setting goals and working systematically towards achieving them, mirroring the goal-setting approach DeCola employs in other areas of his recovery. This goal-oriented framework in therapy helps him track his progress, celebrate achievements, and adjust strategies as needed, contributing to a sense of forward momentum and efficacy in his recovery journey.

In essence, DeCola's engagement with professional mental health support is a cornerstone of his recovery, providing him with expert guidance, effective coping strategies, and a broader perspective on his experiences. This professional support complements his efforts and the support he receives from his community, creating a comprehensive support system that underpins his resilience and promotes sustained progress on his path to well-being.

DeCola's Boundary Setting

DeCola's journey toward mental health recovery is significantly supported by his ability to set healthy boundaries in both his personal and professional life. Mastering this skill allows him to safeguard his emotional energy, ensuring that he remains centered and focused on his recovery and overall well-being. The act of setting boundaries is crucial for DeCola, as it helps him navigate his interactions and commitments in a way that prioritizes his mental health needs.

In his personal life, DeCola learns to communicate his needs and limits unmistakably to friends and family. This clarity helps prevent misunderstandings and ensures that his relationships are supportive and not draining. For instance, by politely declining invitations when he needs time for self-care or therapy, DeCola ensures that he is not spreading himself too thin. This ability to say "no" when necessary is empowering and respects his need for rest and rejuvenation, which are critical for his recovery.

Professionally, setting boundaries involves DeCola being mindful of his workload and stress levels. He learns to negotiate his responsibilities, seeking adjustments or support when tasks become overwhelming. This might involve requesting extensions for deadlines or delegating tasks when possible. By doing so, DeCola avoids the pitfall of overextension, which could lead to burnout—a state that would be detrimental to his mental health recovery.

Boundary setting also extends to DeCola's engagement with digital and social media, where he sets limits to reduce information overload and potential stressors. This might involve designated "unplugged" times, where he disconnects from digital devices to engage more fully with the present moment and his immediate environment. This practice helps maintain his mental clarity and reduces the risk of becoming overwhelmed by the constant barrage of information and social demands.

Furthermore, establishing healthy boundaries allows DeCola to cultivate a sense of autonomy and control over his environment. This sense of control is essential for his self-esteem and agency, reinforcing his belief in his ability to manage his life in a way that supports his mental health. It also fosters an environment where DeCola can grow and thrive, as it minimizes unnecessary stressors that could hinder his progress.

The process of setting and maintaining boundaries also involves continuous self-reflection and adjustment. DeCola learns to assess situations and relationships regularly, making changes to his boundaries as his needs and circumstances evolve. This dynamic approach ensures that his boundaries remain relevant and effective, supporting his well-being in the long term.

In essence, DeCola's ability to set and maintain healthy boundaries is a vital component of his mental health recovery. It enables him to protect his emotional energy, prevent overextension and burnout, and maintain a focus on his well-being. Through this practice, DeCola enhances his resilience, ensuring that he has the strength and stability to continue his path to recovery.

DeCola's Community Engagement

DeCola's active participation in community activities and support groups plays a pivotal role in his mental health recovery. By immersing himself in environments where he can connect with individuals who share similar interests or experiences, DeCola cultivates a sense of belonging that is fundamental to his sense of identity and well-being. This engagement in communal settings offers him not just companionship but also a wealth of support, learning opportunities, and sources of inspiration that enrich his journey toward recovery.

Being part of community activities allows DeCola to step outside of himself and contribute to something larger, which can be incredibly therapeutic and fulfilling. Whether it's volunteering, joining a hobby group, or participating in community service projects, these activities provide a productive outlet for his energies and talents. They also offer a sense of achievement and purpose, reinforcing his value within the community and boosting his self-esteem.

Involvement in support groups specifically tailored to his recovery journey offers DeCola a safe space to share his experiences and challenges with others who truly understand. This mutual sharing and support system is invaluable, as it provides both practical advice for dealing with specific issues and emotional support that comes from knowing he's not alone in his struggles. The solidarity found within these groups fosters a strong sense of belonging and acceptance, crucial elements in the healing process.

Engaging with like-minded individuals in these settings also exposes DeCola to diverse perspectives and coping strategies. He learns from the experiences of others, gaining insights and tools that he can adapt to his own life. This exchange of knowledge and strategies is a dynamic process that contributes to his personal growth and resilience, offering new ways to approach challenges and navigate his recovery.

Furthermore, community engagement often leads to the formation of meaningful relationships that extend beyond the confines of organized activities or meetings. Friendships forged in these contexts are built on shared experiences and mutual understanding, providing a reliable support network. These relationships enrich DeCola's social life and offer him a sense of security, knowing he has people he can turn to in times of need.

Participation in community activities and support groups also keeps DeCola connected to a broader narrative of recovery and growth, reminding him that personal transformation is possible and that change is a collective journey, not a solitary endeavor. Witnessing the progress and victories of others within these communities can be incredibly inspiring, fueling his motivation and hope for the future.

In essence, DeCola's engagement with community activities and support groups is a cornerstone of his mental health recovery. It provides him with a sense of belonging, additional layers of support, and a rich source of inspiration and learning. Through these communal connections, DeCola finds not just solace and understanding but also the strength and encouragement needed to continue his path toward healing and well-being.

DeCola's Flexibility and Adaptability

DeCola's conscious effort to embrace flexibility and adaptability significantly contributes to his mental health recovery, shaping a resilience that is not just robust but also dynamic, allowing him to navigate the ebbs and flows of life with grace. This approach to change and uncertainty is not about passive acceptance but about actively engaging with the unfolding realities of life, prepared to adjust and recalibrate as circumstances evolve.

By cultivating flexibility, DeCola learns to let go of rigid expectations and fixed outcomes, understanding that such attachments can lead to unnecessary stress and disappointment. This openness to different possibilities allows him to approach situations with a curious and open mind rather than with apprehension or resistance. When plans go awry or unexpected challenges arise, he is more likely to view them as opportunities for learning and growth rather than as insurmountable obstacles.

Adaptability, a close ally to flexibility, empowers De-Cola to adjust his strategies and responses based on the demands of the situation. This capability is crucial in his recovery journey, as mental health challenges often require a nuanced and personalized approach. By being adaptable, De-Cola can experiment with various coping strategies and support mechanisms, retaining what works and discarding what doesn't, thus tailoring his recovery path to best suit his evolving needs.

This mindset of flexibility and adaptability also enhances DeCola's problem-solving skills. Faced with change or adversity, he is more likely to think creatively and explore a range of solutions rather than feeling stuck or overwhelmed. This proactive stance not only helps him address immediate challenges but also builds his confidence in handling future uncertainties.

Moreover, embracing change and remaining open enrich DeCola's life, exposing him to diverse perspectives and
opportunities for personal growth. This exposure broadens
his understanding of the world and himself, contributing to
a more rounded and resilient sense of self. It reinforces the
idea that change is an integral part of life and personal development, not something to be feared or avoided.

Furthermore, DeCola's flexibility and adaptability foster
a sense of empowerment and control over his recovery journey. Recognizing that he can adjust his course as needed
gives him a sense of agency, reducing feelings of helplessness that can accompany mental health struggles. This sense
of control is vital for maintaining motivation and hope in the
face of adversity.

In essence, DeCola's commitment to being flexible and
adaptable forms a core component of his mental health recovery. This dynamic approach to resilience enables him to
embrace life's uncertainties with confidence and openness,
ready to learn from every experience. It equips him with the
skills to navigate change effectively, transforming potential
stressors into avenues for growth and strengthening his capacity to thrive in a constantly changing world.

DeCola's Self-Compassion and Forgiveness

DeCola's engagement with self-compassion and forgiveness plays a transformative role in his mental health recovery, infusing his journey with a nurturing and healing energy. By practicing self-compassion, DeCola learns to extend the same kindness and understanding to himself that he would offer to a dear friend. This approach is particularly crucial during moments of setback or when he faces personal challenges. Instead of succumbing to harsh self-criticism or self-doubt, DeCola reminds himself that imperfection and mistakes are inherent aspects of human experience. This gentle and empathetic self-dialogue helps to alleviate the weight of self-imposed pressure and expectations, making it easier for him to navigate through difficult times with grace and patience.

Furthermore, self-compassion encourages DeCola to acknowledge and honor his feelings without judgment or suppression. This acknowledgment fosters emotional healing, as it allows him to process and release negative emotions more effectively. It cultivates an inner environment where self-growth can occur, free from the paralyzing effects of self-criticism. By treating himself with compassion,

DeCola nurtures his self-esteem and reinforces his intrinsic worth, irrespective of external achievements or failures.

Forgiveness, both towards himself and others complements DeCola's practice of self-compassion by releasing the burdens of resentment, anger, and bitterness. Holding onto these negative emotions can be draining and can create emotional barriers that impede recovery and personal growth. DeCola recognizes that forgiveness is not about condoning hurtful actions or denying pain but about freeing himself from the toxic ties that bind him to past grievances. By choosing to forgive, he allows himself to let go of lingering negativity that could hinder his healing process.

Forgiving himself is particularly crucial in DeCola's journey. It involves accepting his past actions and decisions with understanding and empathy rather than dwelling in regret or self-reproach. This self-forgiveness is a powerful act of self-liberation that paves the way for genuine self-improvement and change. It reinforces the idea that he is not defined by his past mistakes but by his capacity for growth and renewal.

Both self-compassion and forgiveness are rooted in a deep understanding of the complexities of human nature and the challenges of life. These practices cultivate an inner strength and flexibility that enhance DeCola's resilience. They teach him to navigate life's inevitable ups and downs with a kinder, more forgiving perspective towards himself and others.

In essence, DeCola's commitment to self-compassion and forgiveness is integral to his mental health recovery. These practices foster a nurturing internal environment conducive to healing, growth, and well-being. By embracing self-compassion and forgiveness, DeCola not only accelerates his recovery but also builds a foundation for a more fulfilling life.

DeCola's Creative Expression

DeCola's engagement with creative expression significantly enhances his mental health recovery, serving as both a therapeutic outlet and a means of reinforcing his sense of identity and resilience. By channeling his experiences and emotions into writing, painting, music, or other creative endeavors, DeCola accesses a profound mode of self-exploration and communication that transcends conventional language.

Writing, for instance, allows DeCola to articulate his thoughts and feelings with clarity and depth. Whether through journaling, poetry, or storytelling, the act of putting pen to paper provides him with a reflective space to process his emotions and experiences. This practice can be particularly cathartic, as it enables him to externalize and examine complex emotions, thereby gaining insights and finding closure in certain aspects of his recovery journey.

Painting and other visual arts offer DeCola a different but equally powerful form of expression. Through color, shape, and texture, he communicates feelings and ideas that might be difficult to articulate verbally. The act of creating visual art becomes a meditative process, where DeCola can lose himself in the flow of creation, experiencing moments of profound peace and focus. This immersion in the creative process can be a significant source of relief from anxiety and stress, providing a refreshing break from the cognitive demands of everyday life.

Music, whether playing an instrument or composing, is another avenue through which DeCola explores and expresses his emotional world. The rhythms, melodies, and harmonies offer a unique language for conveying moods and sentiments, allowing him to connect with his inner self on a deep level. Engaging with music can evoke a wide range of emotions, from joy and nostalgia to sorrow and hope, facilitating an emotional release that is both healing and uplifting.

These creative practices serve not only as outlets for DeCola's emotions but also as tools for self-discovery and personal growth. Through creative expression, he uncovers aspects of himself that may have been suppressed or unrecognized, thereby gaining a fuller understanding of his identity. This process of exploration and self-revelation strengthens his sense of self, contributing to his resilience in the face of life's challenges.

Moreover, the act of creating something tangible—a piece of writing, a painting, a musical composition—reinforces DeCola's sense of agency and accomplishment. Each creative work stands as a testament to his ability to transform thoughts and feelings into something meaningful and beautiful, enhancing his self-efficacy and confidence.

In essence, DeCola's engagement with creative expression is a vital component of his mental health recovery. It provides him with therapeutic outlets for processing emotions, serves as a medium for self-discovery, and reinforces his identity and resilience. Through the act of creation, De-Cola not only navigates his recovery journey more effectively but also enriches his life with a deeper sense of purpose and fulfillment.

DeCola's Humor and Playfulness

In DeCola's life, humor is woven through every thread, a constant, vibrant streak of color even in the darkest of times. His journey through mental health challenges, a path fraught with shadows and storms, saw his humor not just endure but evolve, becoming a beacon of light guiding him toward healing.

Imagine humor as DeCola's loyal companion, one that stuck by him through thick and thin. Even as he navigated the tumultuous waters of his mental health crisis, this companion remained steadfast, a source of relief and resilience. But as DeCola journeyed through the storm, something remarkable happened: his humor transformed, mirroring the changes within him.

Gone were the days of humor that danced on the edges of absurdity, where laughter was a wild, untamed force. As DeCola faced his challenges head-on, his sense of humor matured, shedding its rough edges to reveal a more refined, thoughtful nature. It became a tool not just for amusement but for connection, a way to bridge gaps and build under-standing.

This refined humor became a reflection of DeCola's growth. It was no longer just about eliciting a quick laugh; it was about crafting moments of joy that resonated on a deeper level, humor that was inclusive, uplifting, and, above all, meaningful. It was as if, in the crucible of his struggles, De-Cola had distilled the essence of true humor, one that heals and brings people together.

As DeCola emerged from his mental health crisis, his refined sense of humor became a testament to his journey. It was a humor that acknowledged the complexity of life, that could find light in darkness without diminishing the gravity of the experience. This evolution of humor was not just a personal triumph for DeCola but a gift to those around him, offering laughter that was both a balm and a bond, a gentle reminder of the power of resilience and the enduring strength of a well-timed laugh.

DeCola's appreciation for humor and playfulness signif-icantly enhances his mental health recovery, serving as vital coping mechanisms that infuse his journey with moments of joy and light-heartedness. Recognizing the therapeutic value of laughter and the liberating nature of play, DeCola incorporates these elements into his daily life, discovering that they have the power to transform his outlook and alleviate the weight of his challenges.

Humor, for DeCola, acts as a lens through which the absurdities and contradictions of life can be viewed with a lighter heart. By finding humor in difficult situations, he can create a psychological distance from his problems, making them seem less intimidating. This ability to laugh, even in the face of adversity, DeCola attests, disrupts the cycle of negative thoughts and provides a refreshing perspective that can make challenges more manageable. The act of laughing itself has physiological benefits, including stress reduction, pain relief and muscle relaxation, further aiding his recovery process.

Playfulness, an extension of humor, allows DeCola to engage with the world curiously and imaginatively, reminiscent of the unbridled joy and creativity often seen in childhood. This might involve spontaneous adventures, engaging in playful activities, or simply adopting a more light-hearted approach to daily tasks. Embracing playfulness helps De-

Cola break free from the rigid patterns of thought and behavior that can accompany mental health struggles, fostering a sense of freedom and spontaneity.

Incorporating humor and playfulness into interactions with others also strengthens DeCola's social connections, as shared laughter and joyful experiences create bonds and enhance feelings of camaraderie. These positive social interactions are crucial for his emotional support network, providing him with a sense of belonging and mutual understanding that is essential for his recovery.

Furthermore, humor and playfulness contribute to DeCola's resilience by building his capacity to cope with uncertainty and change. By maintaining a sense of humor and an ability to find joy in small moments, he cultivates a flexible and adaptive mindset that is better equipped to handle life's ups and downs. This resilience is characterized by a buoyant spirit that remains hopeful, even amid difficulty.

In essence, DeCola's embrace of humor and playfulness is a cornerstone of his mental health recovery. These elements serve as powerful coping mechanisms that lighten his emotional load, provide physiological and psychological relief, and strengthen his social bonds. Through laughter and play, DeCola not only navigates his recovery journey with greater ease but also enriches his life with a deeper sense of joy and resilience.

By embracing these additional strategies, DeCola builds a multi-dimensional and robust resilience, empowering him to navigate his recovery with grace, strength, and a deepened capacity for personal growth and transformation.

Chapter 9: The Power of De-Cola's Community

As DeCola steps into the embrace of support groups, he finds himself in a mosaic of stories and souls, each reflecting facets of struggle and resilience that mirror his own. These situations, marked by the raw honesty and vulnerability of the participants, become sanctuaries where the unspeakable can be shared without fear of judgment. Listening to others articulate their battles, DeCola discovers a sense of belonging that had long eluded him, a realization that a robust mental recovery journey is not a solitary one.

DeCola and Others Share Experiences

In DeCola's journey towards mental health recovery, the shared experiences within his support group play a crucial role. This environment, characterized by openness and vulnerability, allows DeCola and others to discuss their struggles and achievements freely. In doing so, DeCola discovers a community where his experiences are mirrored in the stories of others, helping him recognize that his challenges are not solitary battles but part of a broader human experience.

The act of sharing and listening creates a profound sense of belonging among group members. DeCola, who once may have felt isolated by his mental health struggles, finds comfort in knowing that others have walked similar paths. This realization brings a sense of camaraderie and solidarity, making the journey less daunting. The group's collective understanding and empathy make it a sanctuary where DeCola feels seen and heard without judgment.

Moreover, the shared narratives within the group serve as a powerful tool for validation. Hearing others articulate feelings and experiences like his own helps DeCola acknowledge and accept his emotions, fostering a healthier relationship with himself. This validation is a critical step in recovery, as it encourages individuals to confront and address their issues rather than dismissing or suppressing them.

Furthermore, the support group's culture of sharing success stories and coping strategies provides DeCola with practical insights and hope. Witnessing the progress of others instills a belief in the possibility of recovery and motivates him to persevere through difficult times. The exchange of personal triumphs and effective coping mechanisms not only educates but also inspires DeCola, reinforcing the idea that recovery is attainable.

In essence, the shared experiences within DeCola's support group cultivate a nurturing environment that promotes healing and growth. This collective journey of sharing struggles and victories fosters a deep sense of community, understanding, and mutual support, all of which are fundamental to DeCola's path to mental health recovery.

The Emotional Connection of DeCola's Community

DeCola's mental health recovery is significantly bolstered by the emotional connections he forms within his support community. These connections go beyond mere acquaintances, evolving into deep, meaningful relationships with individuals who have an intimate understanding of what it means to navigate mental health challenges. This shared understanding creates a foundation for genuine empathy and connection, making each interaction within the community rich with significance.

Through regular meetings and shared activities, these emotional connections are nurtured and strengthened. Each gathering serves as an opportunity for DeCola and his peers to share not only their struggles but also their joys, fears, and hopes. This continuous exchange fosters a sense of camaraderie and mutual trust, which is crucial for creating an environment where individuals feel safe to express their most vulnerable selves.

The collective pursuit of wellness that DeCola and his community members engage in further cement these bonds. Working together towards a common goal creates a sense of solidarity and shared purpose, making each person's journey feel supported by the collective strength of the group. This dynamic is particularly empowering for DeCola, as it amplifies his sense of agency in his recovery process.

Moreover, these emotional connections provide DeCola with a sense of emotional security. Knowing that he has a network of individuals who not only understand but also care about his well-being gives him a safety net to fall back on during difficult times. This reassurance is invaluable, as it mitigates feelings of isolation and despair that often accompany mental health struggles.

The sense of belonging that DeCola experiences within this community is another critical aspect of his recovery. Feeling part of a group where his experiences are validated and his presence valued helps to rebuild his self-esteem and sense of identity, which mental health issues can erode. This sense of belonging is a powerful antidote to the alienation that often accompanies mental health challenges, fostering a positive self-image and a more hopeful outlook on life.

In sum, the emotional connections DeCola forms within his support community play a central role in his recovery. These connections, characterized by deep understanding, trust, and shared purpose, provide him with emotional security, a sense of belonging, and a robust support system. Together, they create a nurturing environment that significantly contributes to his journey toward healing and well-being.

DeCola's Community Building a Supportive Network

DeCola's mental health recovery is significantly bolstered by the supportive network that extends beyond the confines of his formal support group. This expansive network, encompassing informal gatherings, online forums, and various social activities, plays a crucial role in providing him with a sustained sense of community and belonging.

The informal gatherings, often characterized by casual meetups, coffee chats, or walks in the park, offer DeCola a relaxed environment where connections can deepen outside the structured setting of support group meetings. These gatherings allow for more spontaneous and personal interactions, fostering friendships that are not solely defined by shared challenges but also by the myriad of other interests and experiences that make up DeCola's life. This blend of shared understanding and broader social interaction enriches DeCola's social fabric, providing a more nuanced support system that caters to various aspects of his personality and interests.

Online forums present another layer of support, offering DeCola access to a wide community at any time. These digital platforms become invaluable, especially during times when face-to-face interactions are not possible or when DeCola seeks advice, encouragement, or simply a listening ear outside regular meeting hours. The anonymity and accessibility of online forums can sometimes make it easier to share deeply personal thoughts and questions, broadening the scope of support available to him.

Participation in social activities, whether they are group outings, sports, hobby clubs, or community service projects, introduces DeCola to new experiences and individuals who may not be part of his immediate mental health support circle. Engaging in activities that are enjoyable and fulfilling contributes to a positive sense of self and well-being, offering a respite from the introspection that often accompanies recovery. These activities not only serve as a source of joy and relaxation but also as opportunities to build a diverse network of relationships based on shared interests, further expanding his support system.

This multifaceted network serves as a buffer against isolation, a common challenge in the journey of mental health recovery. The varied points of connection ensure that DeCola has access to support in multiple forms and from different quarters, providing a safety net that is both broad and deep. The sense of belonging and community that comes from this network is a powerful antidote to loneliness, reinforcing DeCola's sense of connectedness and shared humanity.

In essence, the supportive network that DeCola builds around himself, encompassing both structured and informal elements, is instrumental in his recovery. It offers a continuous source of companionship, understanding, and engagement, enriching his social life and providing a comprehensive buffer against the isolation that can impede mental health recovery. This network, with its diverse avenues for connection and support, ensures that DeCola's journey toward healing is both communal and enriched by a wide range of experiences and relationships.

Support Offered by DeCola's Community

As DeCola navigates his path toward mental health recovery, an evolution occurs where he transitions from being predominantly a receiver of support to also becoming a provider of support to others, particularly to newer members of his group. This shift marks a significant milestone in his journey, imbuing him with a newfound sense of empowerment and purpose.

The act of offering support to others allows DeCola to reflect on his journey and recognize the strides he has made in his recovery. This reflection not only consolidates his learning but also highlights his growth, making it more tangible. Being able to share his experiences, insights, and the coping strategies that worked for him with others who are perhaps where he once affirmed the progress he has made. This validation is incredibly empowering and serves as a reminder of his capabilities and resilience.

Furthermore, this role of supporting others fosters a deep sense of fulfillment and purpose in DeCola. Contributing positively to someone else's journey provides him with a meaningful outlet to channel his experiences and lessons learned. The knowledge that his actions and words could potentially lighten someone else's burden or illuminate their path contributes significantly to his sense of self-worth. It reinforces the idea that his experiences, even the challenging ones, hold value not just for him but for others as well.

Moreover, engaging in the act of support allows DeCola to step outside of his challenges and view his situation from a different perspective. This shift in focus can be therapeutic, as it provides a break from his struggles, allowing him to engage in selfless acts that are known to boost mental well-being. The positive feedback and gratitude he receives from those he helps further enhance his self-esteem and sense of accomplishment.

This dynamic of giving and receiving support also strengthens DeCola's connection to the community, reminding him that recovery is not just an individual journey but a communal effort. It highlights the cyclical nature of support within the group, where today's recipients become tomorrow's givers, creating a robust ecosystem of mutual aid and empathy.

In essence, DeCola's role in offering support to others becomes a pivotal aspect of his recovery. It enriches his journey with a sense of empowerment, purpose, and fulfillment, positively impacting his mental well-being. This reciprocal exchange not only aids in his recovery but also fortifies the collective resilience and solidarity of the group, illustrating the profound impact of shared support in the realm of mental health recovery.

Learning and Growth of DeCola's Community

DeCola's path to mental health recovery is significantly enriched by the learning and growth he experiences through the diverse tapestry of backgrounds and experiences represented in his support group. Each member, coming from a unique walk of life, contributes a piece of wisdom or a perspective that DeCola might not have encountered otherwise. This collective pool of knowledge becomes a fertile ground for DeCola's personal development, offering him a broader view of what it means to navigate and manage mental health.

The array of coping strategies, personal anecdotes, and insights shared within the group meetings illuminate various approaches to self-care and mental health management. DeCola, by engaging with these shared experiences, discovers alternative methods and philosophies that challenge and expand his preconceptions. This exposure is crucial, as it encourages him to experiment with new techniques and integrate them into his self-care regimen, thereby enhancing his ability to manage his mental health more effectively.

Moreover, the group's collective wisdom does more than just introduce DeCola to new strategies; it also fosters a deeper understanding of his mental health. Through discussions and exchanges, he learns to recognize patterns, triggers, and coping mechanisms that are more suited to his personal needs and circumstances. This heightened self-awareness is a key component of DeCola's growth, as it empowers him to make more informed decisions about his well-being.

The learning environment within the group also promotes a mindset of continuous personal development. Witnessing the progress of others and sharing in their journey motivates DeCola to remain committed to his growth. The supportive atmosphere encourages him to set personal goals, celebrate achievements, and view setbacks as opportunities for learning rather than as failures.

Additionally, this ongoing learning and growth contribute to DeCola's resilience. Armed with a broader arsenal of coping strategies and a deeper understanding of mental health, he becomes better equipped to face future challenges. This resilience is bolstered by the knowledge that he has a supportive community behind him, ready to share their wisdom and experiences.

In essence, the learning and growth DeCola experiences within his support group play a pivotal role in his mental health recovery. The diverse perspectives and collective wisdom of the group not only broaden his understanding of mental health but also enrich his personal development and enhance his coping strategies. This dynamic environment of shared learning fosters a sense of empowerment and resilience, crucial elements in DeCola's journey toward well-being.

DeCola's Community Fostering a Sense of Purpose

DeCola's involvement in aiding others and contributing to his community plays a transformative role in his mental health recovery, imbuing his life with a profound sense of purpose. This evolution in his role, from being primarily a recipient of support to becoming a source of encouragement and guidance for others, marks a significant phase in his journey, enriching his experience of healing and personal growth.

The act of helping others allows DeCola to step into a role where his experiences, once sources of pain and struggle, become invaluable tools for aiding others. This recontextualization of his experiences gives them new meaning and value, not just as memories of hardship but as beacons of hope for those still navigating the tumultuous waters of their mental health challenges. It underscores the idea that even the most difficult experiences can be transformed into something positive and impactful.

Furthermore, this newfound sense of purpose provides DeCola with a powerful antidote to feelings of aimlessness or despair that often accompany mental health struggles. Engaging in acts of support and community contribution offers him clear and meaningful goals, directing his energy towards constructive and fulfilling endeavors. The satisfaction and fulfillment derived from seeing the positive impact of his efforts on others' lives reinforce his sense of self-worth and accomplishment.

Moreover, DeCola's role as a source of support fosters a deeper connection to his community, creating a sense of belonging and solidarity. This connection is crucial, as it not only provides him with a supportive network but also embeds him within a larger narrative of recovery and resilience, where he plays a key role. Being part of this collective journey enhances his sense of identity, moving beyond the individual to embrace a more communal and interconnected sense of self.

Additionally, the gratitude and recognition he receives from those he helps further affirm his value and contributions, reinforcing his belief in his ability to effect positive change. This feedback loop of support, gratitude, and acknowledgment creates a nurturing environment for DeCola's continued growth and recovery, where his efforts are seen, appreciated, and reciprocated.

In essence, DeCola's engagement in helping others and contributing to his community is not just an adjunct to his recovery but a central component that infuses his journey with purpose, meaning, and connection. This role enriches his life, transforming his path of recovery into a journey of empowerment and communal healing, where he stands as a pivotal figure, offering hope and support to others.

DeCola's Community Celebrating Progress Together

The communal celebration of milestones and progress within DeCola's support network plays a pivotal role in his mental health recovery journey. These celebrations, whether they mark small victories or significant achievements, serve as powerful affirmations of the progress each individual, including DeCola, is making. This practice of acknowledging and celebrating each step forward fosters a culture of positivity and encouragement that is vital for sustained recovery.

When DeCola's achievements are celebrated by the community, it not only validates his efforts but also highlights the tangible outcomes of his hard work and perseverance. This validation is incredibly important as it offers concrete evidence of his growth, making the often intangible process of mental health recovery more visible and real. The act of celebration, therefore, becomes a mirror reflecting his journey, allowing him to see how far he has come and the obstacles he has overcome.

The practice of celebrating progress together also cultivates an environment where success is shared and enjoyed by all, making the recovery journey a communal endeavor rather than an isolated struggle. This collective approach to celebrating progress fosters a strong sense of unity and shared purpose, further enriching the support network's role in DeCola's recovery.

Moreover, these communal celebrations significantly boost morale, not just for DeCola but for the entire group. Witnessing someone else's progress and celebrating it together generates a wave of collective optimism and hope. It's a reminder to all members that progress is possible and that their individual and collective efforts are bearing fruit. This shared joy and optimism are infectious, elevating the group's morale and strengthening the bonds between its members.

In essence, the communal celebration of progress and milestones within DeCola's support network is a cornerstone of his recovery journey. It provides validation, boosts morale, motivates continued effort, and reinforces the communal spirit of the recovery process. These celebrations are not just about acknowledging where one has been but also about looking forward with hope and determination to the road ahead.

In conclusion, the Power of Community is an indispensable component of DeCola's mental health journey. The support group and broader community not only offer a foundation of shared understanding and mutual support but also empower DeCola to contribute positively to the lives of others. This reciprocal dynamic fosters a deep sense of connection and purpose, which is vital for his continued growth and recovery.

Chapter 10: The New Normal

For DeCola, the term "new normal" signifies a profound transformation in his reality following his journey through mental health challenges. This new normal emerged from the considerable changes necessitated by his struggles and recovery, marking a departure from his previous life expectations and behaviors. In Chapter 10: The New Normal, we delve into how DeCola's life has been fundamentally altered, with shifts in his daily routines, interactions, and self-perception becoming permanent fixtures. This chapter explores how DeCola has adjusted to these changes, embracing resilience and innovation to navigate a world that looks markedly different from his past. It highlights how these adaptations have not only helped him cope but have also opened up new ways of relating to others and understanding his place in a reshaped world. Through DeCola's story, we see how a new normal can be both challenging and enriching, providing fresh foundations on which to build a future.

DeCola Integrates Self-Acceptance

In his journey toward mental health recovery, DeCola reaches a pivotal moment of integrated self-acceptance, where he recognizes his mental health challenges as part of his broader identity without letting them define him entirely. This nuanced understanding marks a significant shift in how he views himself and his experiences, offering a more compassionate and comprehensive perspective on his life.

This integrated self-acceptance begins with DeCola acknowledging the reality of his mental health condition and facing it without denial or shame. By doing so, he takes an important step toward understanding that while his mental health is an integral part of his life's narrative, it is not the entirety of his story. This realization helps him to see himself as a multifaceted individual with a wide range of attributes, experiences, and aspirations beyond his mental health challenges.

Moreover, DeCola's journey of acceptance involves dismantling the internalized stigma often associated with mental health issues. He learns to challenge and discard the societal misconceptions and prejudices that can infiltrate one's self-perception, replacing them with a narrative of strength, resilience, and complexity. This process is crucial for fostering a healthier self-view, as it allows DeCola to appreciate the full scope of his identity without judgment or self-reproach.

Integrated self-acceptance also empowers DeCola to openly communicate about his mental health with others, contributing to a broader culture of transparency and understanding. By sharing his experiences without fear of stigma, he not only bolsters his sense of self but also encourages others to view mental health as a natural part of the human experience, deserving of empathy and respect.

Furthermore, this acceptance enriches DeCola's relationships with others. It enables him to engage more authentically, free from the masks and defenses that might have previously shielded his vulnerabilities. This authenticity fosters deeper connections and a stronger support network, which are invaluable resources in his ongoing recovery.

In essence, integrated self-acceptance is a cornerstone of DeCola's mental health recovery, providing a foundation for a more balanced and fulfilling life. By embracing his mental health as one aspect of his broader identity, DeCola cultivates a sense of wholeness and resilience that supports his journey toward well-being. This acceptance not only benefits him personally but also contributes to a wider societal shift towards a more inclusive and compassionate understanding of mental health.

DeCola's Continuous Care

DeCola's mental health recovery is characterized by an ongoing commitment to continuous care, a journey that challenges the traditional notion of a definitive cure. This aspect of his recovery underscores the dynamic nature of mental well-being, where management and care are not static but evolve in response to life's changes and personal growth.

Recognizing the necessity of continuous care, DeCola adopts a proactive approach to his mental health, understanding that his needs will fluctuate over time due to various factors such as stress, life transitions, and personal development. This realization leads him to regularly engage in self-assessment, taking stock of his emotional state, coping mechanisms, and overall well-being. These periodic check-ins allow DeCola to identify areas that may require additional attention or adjustment in his care strategies, ensuring that his approach remains responsive and tailored to his current circumstances.

Moreover, DeCola's commitment to continuous care involves a diverse range of practices that cater to different aspects of his mental health. This includes therapy sessions that provide professional guidance and support, medication management when necessary, and self-care activities that nurture his emotional, physical, and spiritual well-being. By integrating these practices into his daily routine, DeCola creates a comprehensive care plan that addresses his needs holistically.

DeCola's journey also highlights the importance of flexibility in mental health management. As his life circumstances and personal insights evolve, so too do his care needs. This requires him to remain open to modifying his care practices, whether that means exploring new therapeutic techniques, adjusting his self-care activities, or seeking different forms of support. This adaptability is crucial for ensuring that his mental health care remains effective and supportive of his overall well-being.

Furthermore, DeCola's approach to continuous care extends beyond individual practices to include the cultivation of a supportive environment that nurtures his mental health. This involves fostering positive relationships, engaging in meaningful activities, and creating a lifestyle that aligns with his values and needs. By surrounding himself with a conducive environment, DeCola reinforces the gains made through his direct care practices, further supporting his journey toward recovery.

In essence, the narrative of DeCola's recovery journey illustrates the critical role of continuous care in managing mental health. By challenging the notion of a one-time cure and embracing an ongoing commitment to self-assessment and adaptable care practices, DeCola navigates the complexities of mental well-being with resilience and self-compassion. This approach not only supports his immediate recovery but also equips him with the skills and mindset to maintain his mental health in the face of future challenges, embodying a sustainable path to well-being.

DeCola's Adaptive Coping Strategies

In DeCola's narrative of mental health recovery, the development and adaptation of coping strategies emerge as key elements that significantly contribute to his journey. This evolution in coping mechanisms underscores the dynamic nature of mental health management, where strategies that prove effective at one stage may need refinement or replacement as circumstances and individual growth dictate.

DeCola's initial foray into coping strategies might have included a set of techniques that addressed his needs at the outset of his recovery. These could have ranged from deep breathing exercises and mindfulness meditation to more structured practices like cognitive-behavioral techniques. Over time, however, DeCola notices shifts in his responses to these strategies. What once offered relief might not yield the same level of efficacy, prompting a reassessment of his approach.

This realization leads DeCola to explore a broader spectrum of coping mechanisms. He becomes open to integrating new practices into his routine, such as engaging in physical activity, which has been shown to alleviate symptoms of stress and anxiety, or embracing creative outlets like writing or art, which offer alternative means of expression and emotional release. The willingness to experiment and embrace new strategies is crucial, as it allows DeCola to discover what resonates with his evolving needs and preferences.

Moreover, DeCola's adaptive approach to coping strategies extends to his social and interpersonal interactions. He learns the value of setting healthy boundaries, seeking support from his social network, and, when necessary, distancing himself from toxic or stressful relationships. These social coping strategies become integral components of his overall approach, highlighting the importance of environmental factors in mental health management.

The process of adapting coping strategies also involves a degree of self-reflection and mindfulness. DeCola becomes adept at recognizing early signs of stress or emotional distress, allowing him to adjust his coping strategies before challenges become overwhelming proactively. This pre-emptive approach not only mitigates potential setbacks but also reinforces DeCola's sense of agency and control over his mental health.

Furthermore, DeCola's journey illustrates the importance of a flexible mindset in the face of change. By accepting that adaptation is a natural and necessary part of growth, he cultivates resilience and a more sustainable approach to managing mental health challenges. This flexibility ensures that his arsenal of coping strategies remains diverse and effective, tailored to meet the unique demands of each phase of his recovery.

In essence, the emphasis on developing and adapting coping strategies within DeCola's mental health recovery narrative highlights the need for a dynamic and responsive approach to mental well-being. By remaining open to new techniques and approaches, DeCola not only navigates his recovery more effectively but also lays a foundation for enduring resilience in the face of life's inevitable stressors and changes.

DeCola's Proactive Support Systems

In DeCola's journey toward mental health recovery, proactive engagement with various support systems plays a pivotal role, serving as a foundational pillar that sustains and propels his progress. This active involvement with therapy, support groups, and community resources creates a robust network of support tailored to meet his evolving needs and circumstances.

Therapy stands as a cornerstone in DeCola's support system, offering a consistent and professional resource for guidance, insight, and therapeutic intervention. By maintaining open and regular communication with his therapist, DeCola ensures that his care is responsive to his current mental health status, allowing for adjustments in therapeutic techniques and focus areas as his journey unfolds. This dynamic relationship with his therapist fosters a safe space for exploration, growth, and healing, where DeCola can address emerging challenges and celebrate progress with a trusted professional.

Support groups provide another layer of proactive support for DeCola, connecting him with individuals who share similar experiences and challenges. These groups offer a sense of community and mutual understanding that is deeply affirming. Through regular participation, DeCola benefits from the collective wisdom, empathy, and encouragement of peers, which bolster his resilience and sense of belonging. The fluid nature of support groups, with members at various stages of their journeys, ensures that the guidance and insights available are both diverse and adaptable to DeCola's changing needs.

Community resources extend DeCola's network of support beyond the confines of formal therapy and support groups, offering a broader array of services and activities that contribute to his well-being. Engaging with community centers, mental health workshops, and wellness activities, DeCola accesses educational materials, skill-building sessions, and recreational opportunities that enhance his quality of life and coping repertoire. These community connections also serve to integrate DeCola more fully into the societal fabric, reducing isolation and reinforcing the notion that he is not alone in his journey.

The proactive nature of DeCola's engagement with these support systems is crucial. Rather than passively receiving assistance, DeCola takes an active role in seeking out and utilizing available resources. This proactive stance not only empowers him to tailor the support he receives to his current needs but also fosters a sense of agency and self-advocacy that is vital for recovery.

Moreover, the adaptability of these support systems is a key feature, providing DeCola with the flexibility to navigate the unpredictable terrain of mental health recovery. As his circumstances, challenges, and achievements evolve, so does the network of support around him, offering reassurance that he has the resources to face both current and future challenges.

In essence, DeCola's proactive engagement with therapy, support groups, and community resources forms an adaptable and multifaceted support network that is instrumental in his mental health recovery. This network not only offers immediate assistance and connection but also empowers DeCola to manage his mental health proactively, contributing to a resilient and hopeful approach to his ongoing journey.

DeCola's Holistic Self-Care

DeCola's mental health recovery is markedly enhanced by his holistic approach to self-care, which recognizes the interconnectivity of physical, emotional, and spiritual well-being. This comprehensive perspective on self-care not only addresses the symptoms of his mental health challenges but also nurtures his overall sense of health and fulfillment.

Physical well-being forms a critical pillar of DeCola's holistic self-care regimen. Regular exercise becomes a keystone habit, providing numerous benefits that extend beyond mere physical health. Physical activity releases endorphins, often referred to as the body's natural mood elevators, which help to alleviate symptoms of stress and depression. Additionally, the discipline and routine of regular exercise instill a sense of accomplishment and structure in DeCola's daily life, reinforcing his agency and self-efficacy.

Nutrition also plays a vital role in DeCola's self-care strategy. Understanding the profound impact of diet on mental health, DeCola makes mindful choices about his food intake, focusing on a balanced diet rich in nutrients that support brain health and emotional stability. This conscious approach to nutrition not only fuels his body optimally but also serves as an act of self-respect and care, reinforcing the value he places on his well-being.

Creative expression emerges as another essential facet of DeCola's holistic self-care practice. Whether through writing, painting, music, or any other creative outlet, DeCola finds a unique and potent way to process and articulate his emotions. These creative endeavors offer him a sense of release and catharsis, allowing him to externalize complex feelings in a constructive and often beautiful form. Moreover, engaging in creative activities provides DeCola with a sense of identity and accomplishment that transcends his mental health challenges, enriching his sense of self.

Spiritual practices, whether they involve organized religion, meditation, mindfulness, or nature walks, become crucial components of DeCola's self-care regimen. These practices offer him a sense of connection to something greater than himself, providing comfort, purpose, and perspective. The peace and introspection gained through spiritual activities foster a deep sense of inner harmony and resilience, anchoring DeCola during times of turmoil and uncertainty.

This holistic approach to self-care, encompassing physical, emotional, and spiritual well-being, equips DeCola with a comprehensive toolkit for managing his mental health. By nurturing his body, mind, and spirit, DeCola ensures that his self-care practices are balanced and integrative, addressing the full spectrum of his needs. This multifaceted approach not only aids in his immediate recovery but also lays the foundation for sustained well-being and resilience, empowering DeCola to lead a fulfilling and balanced life.

DeCola's Spiritual Practices and Reflection

DeCola's spiritual practices are integral to his mental health recovery, offering a profound sense of purpose and connection beyond the tangible aspects of daily life. By dedicating time to meditation, prayer, nature walks, and other spiritual activities, he accesses deeper peace and understanding, which anchor him during challenging times.

Meditation helps DeCola cultivate mindfulness and inner tranquillity. By focusing his attention on the present moment, he quiets his mind, relieving anxiety and stress. This practice enhances his self-awareness and emotional regulation, significantly contributing to his mental well-being.

Prayer reinforces DeCola's sense of hope and guidance. Whether seeking strength, expressing gratitude, or connecting with a higher power, prayer provides a channel of communication that transcends the physical realm. This act of faith offers comfort and reassurance, reminding him he is not alone and that a greater force supports and guides him.

Nature walks ground DeCola in the beauty and serenity of the natural world. Immersing himself in nature provides peace and a reminder of the interconnectedness of all living things. This connection renews his perspective, helping him see his challenges as part of a larger tapestry of life. The simplicity of the natural environment reminds him of life's beauty and the importance of nurturing his relationship with the world around him.

Collectively, these spiritual practices help DeCola understand his place in the universe and his connection to something greater than himself. This sense of belonging offers a solid foundation when facing life's uncertainties, making his spiritual life a powerful source of strength and resilience. The purpose and meaning derived from these practices imbue his life with direction and intentionality, reminding him that his recovery journey is about personal growth and spiritual enlightenment.

In essence, DeCola's commitment to spiritual practices like meditation, prayer, and nature walks is pivotal to his mental health recovery. These activities provide calm, purpose, and connection, offering a stable anchor amidst life's challenges. Through his spiritual practices, DeCola finds solace, strength, and a deeper sense of belonging, expanding his perspective on his journey toward healing and well-being.

Mindfulness and regular self-reflection are also crucial to DeCola's holistic self-care regimen, providing tools to maintain continuous awareness of his mental state. Mindfulness, rooted in being fully present and non-judgmental, helps DeCola observe his thoughts and feelings from a detached perspective, recognizing them as transient. This practice enables him to navigate emotional fluctuations with greater stability, reducing the impact of negative thoughts and feelings. It also enhances his appreciation for everyday experiences, bolstering his resilience against stress and adversity.

Self-reflection complements mindfulness by offering structured moments for introspection and evaluation. Through regular self-reflection, DeCola gains insights into his coping mechanisms, behavioral patterns, and emotional triggers. This ongoing self-assessment allows him to identify areas needing additional support or where current strategies may be ineffective. Reflecting on his experiences, successes, and challenges deepens his understanding of his mental health journey, enabling informed decisions about his care.

Together, mindfulness and self-reflection foster a proactive approach to mental health management. DeCola's heightened awareness of his mental state ensures he remains attuned to subtle shifts in well-being, enabling timely interventions. This proactive stance mitigates the severity of distressing episodes and reinforces his sense of control and agency over his mental health.

Additionally, mindfulness and self-reflection contribute to DeCola's emotional regulation. By recognizing and accepting his emotions without judgment, he navigates emotional turbulence with grace and resilience. This emotional regulation is key to his recovery, reducing the likelihood of being overwhelmed by intense emotions and promoting a balanced mental state.

In summary, integrating mindfulness and self-reflection into DeCola's self-care approach is instrumental in his mental health recovery. These practices cultivate a deep awareness of his mental state, enabling timely interventions and informed adjustments to his care strategies. Through mindfulness and self-reflection, DeCola navigates his recovery with greater insight and resilience, enriching his life with a profound sense of presence and appreciation.

DeCola's Education and Awareness

DeCola's mental health recovery journey is significantly bolstered by an ongoing commitment to education and awareness about mental health issues. This commitment to learning plays a dual role: it not only empowers DeCola with the knowledge to navigate his recovery more effectively but also contributes to broader societal understanding and destigmatization of mental health challenges.

For DeCola, staying informed about various aspects of mental health, including understanding different conditions, recognizing symptoms, and being aware of the latest treatments and therapeutic approaches, becomes an empowering tool. This knowledge enables him to actively participate in discussions with his healthcare providers, making decisions about his care that are informed by both professional advice and his understanding of his needs and options. This collaborative approach to treatment planning increases his sense of agency and satisfaction with his care, as he feels more in control of his recovery journey.

Furthermore, DeCola's exploration of different coping mechanisms and self-care strategies through education allows him to tailor his approach to managing daily stressors and triggers. By learning about a wide array of techniques, from mindfulness and stress reduction to exercise and nutrition, he is able to experiment with and adopt practices that resonate most with his lifestyle and preferences. This personalized approach to self-care enhances the effectiveness of his overall mental health management strategy.

Beyond personal benefits, DeCola's pursuit of mental health education plays a crucial role in combating stigma and misinformation in society. By sharing accurate information and personal insights with his social circle and community, DeCola helps to dispel myths and stereotypes associated with mental illness. His willingness to engage in open conversations about mental health fosters a more inclusive and understanding environment, encouraging others to seek help without fear of judgment.

Moreover, DeCola's commitment to education and awareness extends to advocating for mental health literacy in various settings, from schools and workplaces to social media platforms. By supporting initiatives that promote mental health education, he contributes to creating a culture where mental well-being is prioritized and support is readily available.

In essence, the emphasis on education and awareness in DeCola's mental health recovery narrative highlights the transformative power of knowledge. Staying informed about mental health conditions, treatments, and coping mechanisms not only empowers DeCola to make informed decisions about his care but also enables him to contribute to a more informed and compassionate society. Through education, DeCola not only navigates his recovery with greater confidence and effectiveness but also plays a part in fostering a broader cultural shift toward greater understanding and acceptance of mental health challenges.

DeCola's Lifestyle Integration

DeCola's approach to mental health recovery significantly emphasizes the integration of mental health care into his daily routines and lifestyle choices, mirroring the attention often given to physical health. This seamless incorporation of mental well-being practices into everyday life is not only practical but also transformative, allowing DeCola to maintain a healthier balance and mitigate the risk of burnout.

For DeCola, lifestyle integration means embedding mindfulness practices into the start or end of his day, making them as routine as brushing his teeth or having breakfast. This could involve a few minutes of meditation each morning to set a positive tone for the day or a brief reflective journaling session each night to process the day's events and emotions. These practices become anchors in his daily routine, ensuring that he consistently attends to his mental wellbeing amidst the hustle and bustle of life.

Nutrition and physical activity are also viewed through the lens of mental health care. DeCola understands that a balanced diet and regular exercise are not just about physical fitness but are crucial for mental health. He makes mindful choices about what he eats, focusing on foods known to support brain health and mood stability. Similarly, exercise becomes a non-negotiable part of his routine, valued not only for its physical benefits but also for its proven effectiveness in reducing symptoms of anxiety and depression.

Social interactions and relationships are another area where DeCola integrates mental health care into his lifestyle.

He consciously cultivates positive relationships that support his well-being and actively engages in social activities that bring him joy and relaxation. At the same time, he becomes adept at setting healthy boundaries to protect his mental space, ensuring that his social life nourishes rather than drains his mental energy.

Work and leisure are balanced in a way that prioritizes mental health. DeCola ensures that his work commitments do not overwhelm his capacity, taking breaks when needed and using his leisure time to engage in activities that rejuvenate his mind and spirit. This balance prevents burnout and keeps stress at manageable levels, supporting his overall recovery journey.

Besides, DeCola's approach to lifestyle integration involves regular reflection and adjustment. He remains vigilant about how different aspects of his life impact his mental health, ready to make changes when certain routines or habits no longer serve his well-being. This flexibility is key to maintaining a lifestyle that continuously supports his mental health.

In essence, the integration of mental health care into DeCola's daily routines and lifestyle choices is a cornerstone of his recovery. By making mental well-being a fundamental part of his everyday life, DeCola ensures that his approach to mental health is sustainable and effective. This holistic and integrated approach not only aids in his immediate recovery but also lays the groundwork for long-term resilience and well-being, showcasing the profound impact of lifestyle integration on mental health recovery.

DeCola's Advocacy and Community Engagement

DeCola's mental health recovery journey is significantly enriched by his active involvement in advocacy and engagement with mental health communities. This participation not only bolsters his sense of belonging and purpose but also plays a crucial role in enhancing societal empathy, understanding, and support for mental health issues.

By stepping into the role of an advocate, DeCola transforms his personal experiences with mental health into powerful narratives that can educate, inspire, and motivate change. Whether through public speaking, blogging, social media, or participation in mental health awareness events, DeCola shares his journey openly, shedding light on the realities of living with and recovering from mental health challenges. This transparency helps to dismantle stigma and misconceptions surrounding mental health, fostering a more informed and compassionate societal perspective.

Engagement with mental health communities, both online and in-person, provides DeCola with a robust support network of individuals who share similar experiences and challenges. These communities offer a space for mutual support, where members can exchange coping strategies, celebrate each other's successes, and offer comfort during difficult times. For DeCola, being part of such communities reinforces a sense of belonging and solidarity, reminding him that he is not alone in his journey.

Furthermore, DeCola's involvement in these communities extends beyond seeking support to actively providing it. By offering guidance, sharing resources, and simply being present for others, DeCola contributes to the collective well-being of the community. This reciprocal exchange of support not only aids in his recovery but also enhances his sense of purpose and self-worth.

Community engagement also allows DeCola to stay abreast of the latest developments in mental health care, advocacy, and policy. This continuous learning empowers him to make informed decisions about his care and advocacy efforts, ensuring that his contributions are both relevant and impactful.

Furthermore, DeCola's advocacy and community engagement serve to inspire others who may be struggling in silence. By seeing DeCola take an active role in his recovery and advocacy, others are encouraged to seek help, engage with supportive communities, and perhaps even become advocates themselves. This ripple effect has the potential to foster a more supportive and understanding environment for everyone affected by mental health issues.

In essence, DeCola's advocacy and engagement with mental health communities form an integral part of his recovery process. These activities not only support his healing and growth but also contribute to a larger movement toward societal acceptance and support for mental health. Through advocacy and community engagement, DeCola finds a sense of belonging, purpose, and empowerment, underscoring the profound impact of these endeavors on both individual recovery and broader societal change.

Conclusion: Subscribing to Thrive is Hope in Action

In the resonant conclusion, DeCola's voyage through the landscape of mental health emerges as a profound symbol of hope and unwavering resilience, illuminating the path for those entangled in their mental health struggles. This final chapter skillfully crafts a narrative that pays tribute to the indomitable spirit of humanity, honoring the courage required to face and navigate through the obscure realms of personal fears while celebrating the remarkable strength revealed in embracing one's vulnerabilities.

DeCola's journey, moving from the depths of despair to the bright domains of self-awareness and acceptance, showcases the incredible capacity for change inherent in the human spirit. His story goes beyond the individual, reflecting the collective journey of hardship and victory that many endure in silence. DeCola becomes more than just a protagonist; he becomes a mirror reflecting our shared fears, aspirations, and the continuous quest for peace. His narrative, adorned with challenges and triumphs, serves as a source of comfort and inspiration for those maneuvering through the unpredictable waters of mental health challenges.

344

The story concludes by highlighting a fundamental truth: the complexities of mental health are an integral part of our shared human story, not to be shunned or hidden away in shame. It elevates the act of seeking help to a testament of undeniable bravery, a positive step toward the path of healing and deep self-realization. Through DeCola's journey, the common misconception of mental health as an isolated battle is dispelled, shedding light on the significant role of community support, empathy, and shared experiences in the journey toward healing.

In essence, this closure to DeCola's journey sparks a conversation about the nature of our collective struggle with mental health, advocating for a shift in perspective towards one of understanding, compassion, and collective upliftment.

DeCola's story is one of a heartfelt expedition through the ups and downs of dealing with mental health, designed to enlighten and provide comfort to others on a similar path. The closing chapter of "Subscribed to Thrive" unfolds like a serene aftermath to a tempest, revealing DeCola's quiet yet significant transformation following the tumult of his experiences. It's a comforting finale to the intense narrative of obstacles, revelations, and achievements that populate his tale.

In this final act, we witness DeCola in a state of peace and purposefulness, having transformed the tribulations of his past into a steadfast commitment to advocating for mental health, not just for himself but for all. DeCola has become a guiding light in his community, leading and uplifting others still on their journey to finding their path. This role of advocacy and support emerges naturally from his own experiences, a sincere way to reciprocate the support that once sustained him.

Now, DeCola's days are filled with meaningful engagements, whether facilitating discussions in support groups, participating in mental health education, or simply sharing his journey with others in search of solace in collective stories. Each interaction is characterized by the same empathy and understanding that once made a difference during his bleakest moments. This cycle of giving and receiving creates an environment where mental health is openly discussed, devoid of stigma, and acknowledged as an essential aspect of everyone's journey.

In moments of solitude, DeCola contemplates the journey that led him here—the depths explored, the hurdles surmounted, and the inner fortitude uncovered. These reflections are imbued with gratitude for the growth, the lessons learned, and the connections forged along the way.

"Subscribed to Thrive" is more than just a title; it encapsulates DeCola's philosophy. It signifies a daily recommitment to embrace life in all its complexity, to maintain hope in the face of despair, and to continually prioritize mental health as an act of self-care and survival. This closing chapter emphasizes the notion that choosing to live, truly live, is a decision reaffirmed each day through actions, mindset, and the willingness to both seek and offer support.

DeCola's journey toward full restoration was a mosaic of perseverance, support, and personal growth, culminating in a triumphant re-orientation into his community. This renaissance was not just a return to his pre-crisis state but a rebirth into a more resilient, self-aware individual, enriched by his experiences and the wisdom they imparted.

The cornerstone of DeCola's restoration was the multi-faceted support system that encircled him, a fabric woven from threads of professional care, family support, and community resources. Each element played a distinct role, yet it was their synergy that propelled him forward. Professional therapists equipped him with coping strategies and insights into his mental patterns, while family and friends offered a cushion of emotional support, acceptance, and love. Community resources and support groups connected him with others who shared similar journeys, fostering a sense of belonging and mutual empowerment.

As DeCola heals, he gradually sheds the layers of doubt and isolation that envelop him, revealing a newfound confidence and a desire to engage with the world around him. A series of deliberate steps marked his re-orientation into the community, each taken with a mindful appreciation for the journey and the lessons it had taught him.

One of the most profound shifts in DeCola's restoration was his approach to relationships. Where once he trod cautiously, fearful of misunderstanding and rejection, he now navigates his social interactions with openness and authenticity. This transformation was rooted in his deepened understanding of himself and his mental health journey, allowing him to communicate his needs and boundaries more effectively and to forge connections based on genuine understanding and respect.

DeCola also found solace and purpose in advocacy and volunteering, channels through which he could give back to the community that had supported his recovery. By sharing his story and contributing to mental health awareness initiatives, he not only demystified mental health challenges but also offered hope to those still ensnared in their struggles. This engagement brought a sense of fulfilment and community integration that DeCola had longed for, reinforcing his sense of identity and belonging.

Moreover, DeCola embraced opportunities for lifelong learning and personal development, recognizing that growth was an ongoing process. Whether through formal education, skill-building workshops, or creative pursuits, he continuously sought to expand his horizons, enriching his life and, by extension, the community around him.

DeCola's full restoration and community re-orientation were a testament to the transformative power of resilience, support, and self-compassion. His journey from the depths of a mental health crisis to the heights of community integration and advocacy highlighted the potential for recovery and growth in the face of adversity. DeCola's story became a guiding light of hope, not only for him but for the broader community, illuminating the path toward understanding, acceptance, and mutual support in the collective journey toward mental wellness.

Printed in Great Britain
by Amazon